Survival Strategies for People on the Autism Spectrum

also by Marc Fleisher

Making Sense of the Unfeasible
My Life Journey with Asperger Syndrome
ISBN 1 84310 165 3

of related interest

Asperger's Syndrome
A Guide for Parents and Professionals
Tony Attwood
Foreword by Lorna Wing
ISBN 1 85302 577 1

Build Your Own Life
A Self-Help Guide For Individuals With Asperger Syndrome
Wendy Lawson
ISBN 1 84310 114 9

**How to Find Work that Works for People
with Asperger Syndrome**
The Ultimate Guide for Getting People with Asperger
Syndrome into the Workplace (and keeping them there!)
Gail Hawkins
ISBN 1 84310 151 3

Pretending to be Normal
Living with Asperger's Syndrome
Liane Holliday Willey
Foreword by Tony Attwood
ISBN 1 85302 749 9

Survival Strategies for People on the Autism Spectrum

Marc Fleisher

Jessica Kingsley Publishers
London and Philadelphia

First published in 2006
by Jessica Kingsley Publishers
116 Pentonville Road
London N1 9JB, UK
and
400 Market Street, Suite 400
Philadelphia, PA 19106, USA

www.jkp.com

Library of Congress Cataloging in Publication Data
Fleisher, Marc, 1967-
Survival strategies for people on the autism spectrum / Marc Fleisher.
    p. cm.
Includes index.
ISBN-13: 978-1-84310-261-8 (pbk. : alk. paper)
    ISBN-10: 1-84310-261-7 (pbk. : alk. paper) 1. Autism in children. 2. Autism in
children--Rehabilitation. I. Title.
RJ506.A9F59 2005
618.92'85882--dc22

                                                    2005011554

British Library Cataloguing in Publication Data
A CIP catalogue record for this book is available from the British Library

ISBN-13: 978 1 84310 261 8
ISBN-10: 1 84310 261 7

Printed and Bound in Great Britain by
Athenaeum Press, Gateshead, Tyne and Wear

This book is dedicated to Sheila Coates, both for her considerable help in its construction, and for her infinite help to autism in general

Acknowledgements

Maurice Fleisher
Sheila Coates
Rebecca Fraser
Ruth Smith
Rosemary West
Margaret Shapley and family
Daphne Fawcett
Kristen Aldridge
Emma Selleck
Eva Williams and family
Hilary Rifkin
Kathy Erangey
Pavanne Chatha
Sham Chatha
June Wise and family
Lesley Hatton
Beverly Williams
Vivien Izzard

Contents

Introduction

This book represents my second publication on autism to be released, following my autobiography *Making Sense of the Unfeasible*, also published by Jessica Kingsley Publishers, in June 2003. Before I discuss the aims and layout of this book, a brief review of my former work is in order. For those readers amongst you who have already read my autobiography, this will serve to jog your memories of the key points in my life story; for others who have perhaps never heard of me, it will provide a general outline of the type of person who is writing. My autobiography attempted to explain not only actual physical occurrences at different stages of my life, but also my inner personal and mental feelings.

I was born on 3 May 1967 in Bury St Edmunds in Suffolk and lived in an average-sized family home in Pakenham with my mother and father and one sister, slightly older than me. In my early childhood years I often felt lonely and very isolated from other children of my age, and had virtually no interest in interaction with the others, preferring to withdraw into my own fantasy world of obsessions and rituals. When I was about five, my parents, who had not been able to pinpoint the nature of my difficulties, took me to see a young, inexperienced junior doctor, who promptly labelled me as mentally retarded and beyond hope of any progress. As a further blow a few years later, my only sister was tragically killed in a car crash while we were abroad. This served to intensify my acute anxiety about things greatly when I was trying to cope with the resulting grief, as well as with my disability.

Shortly after this, we moved house to High Wycombe, and at the age of 11 I was referred to a brilliant doctor in London, who within a few minutes diagnosed me with having Asperger's Syndrome. This was a huge relief to my parents, who now not only knew why I was finding many things difficult, both socially and practically, but could also now start looking for professional help. I started receiving this from the Chinnor Resource Unit for autistic youngsters, at which the staff were all thoroughly trained in the condition. Through this assistance I started making substantial progress academically and achieved many top grades in my high school exams (at Lord Williams Upper School), but continued to be bullied, teased and victimised, feeling a total outsider on a social front, with virtually no friends.

When I left school in 1985, I managed to hold down a job in the accounts department of a local transport firm for more than three years. I enjoyed the figure work involved, having acquired a taste for mathematics, but normal office deadlines often made me ill with worry. Then, in the most stressful part of my life, my mother fell very ill with cancer. Just a few months before she died I was able to move into my own rented accommodation, having learnt independent skills at a special hostel for young people with learning difficulties shortly beforehand. I had continued to use an imaginary parallel world in my mind, of wars and conflict, to help me cope with difficult and challenging situations, almost like a tortoise retreating into its shell for protection.

When my mother died on 18 May 1991, the situation appeared hopeless, resembling total anarchy, like a nuclear devastation in my parallel land. But somehow, with the combination of social services, loving support from the rest of my family, the earlier foundational skills set by the Chinnor Unit, the hostel, and my own determination, I was able to find strength and come through this terrible period of my life, not just in becoming independent in my own right (requiring only minimum support from rehab services), but also to work for other people in a similar position to live more fulfilling lives as well. Exceeding my mother's wishes of independence for me, I set out on a two-part mission to improve my own confidence and educate others.

Part 1 of my task was to achieve academic excellence, both for my own self-esteem and also to prove to all those bullies who had called me stupid earlier in life that they were wrong, and that I had the ability to set myself a hard and far-reaching goal and to achieve it. This was made possible through aid from social services in gaining a place at Brunel University, a place where I was to study for six years. Being a perfectionist, I believed that I underperformed in my first degree (BSc in mathematics) by getting only a 2:1, so decided to go on and study for a further three years to get my postgraduate degree (in maths also).

The second part of my proposed mission in life was to spread the awareness of autism and Asperger's Syndrome as far as possible into the general population, proving through my own experiences that there need not be any restrictions on what can be achieved. There were a number of ways in which I set about this task, one of these being to give talks about the condition. Becoming a public speaker enabled me to deliver a large number of lectures both in small local events and to youngsters in schools, up to large national and international conferences. I had the chance to appear on national TV, where I featured in the BBC's *QED* programme, and also separately on a local TV station. I became a patron of a local sports club, assisting the coaches to give tennis lessons to youngsters with disabilities. This was a great way of helping and relating to others, while also being involved with the game I had grown to love.

Then more recently I found another way to increase awareness on autism – by writing articles about it and having them published. I started off with small sections of work in local magazines, but worked up to larger items and then decided to write my autobiography. This, then, was chiefly about myself and my experiences to date. For a while I experienced the joy of having my first major book published, but of course the second part of my mission in life has been continuing and I felt I must now carry on working for the common good of progress in autistic research. I now had the inspiration to begin this, my second book.

CHAPTER 1

Summary of Contents and Aims

This book should not be regarded simply as a continuation of my autobiography, for there are a number of important differences in the aims of each. First, although I shall still be relating quite often to my own experiences here, I shall, as a rule, be talking in a more general sense. This work is primarily a guide for other individuals in a similar position to myself on developing strategies to master and cope better with new and challenging situations, chiefly catering for the age range of teenager and above. Parts of the text may also appeal to other readers, in particular Chapter 2 ('An Overview of Autism'), Chapter 4 ('The Vital Role of Communication') and Chapter 5 ('The Art of Independent Living') could be of interest to the parents and associated families of the autistic individual, while Chapter 7 ('Further Education and Training Survival Guide') might also be of interest to social workers, care managers and teachers. Chapter 11 ('Autism in a Nutshell') could also be of interest to all of these latter groups. Second, I shall be studying many aspects in greater depth than I was able to in my autobiography. For example, my discussion on life in further education and training in Chapter 7 will consider the fact that there will be different circumstances for each individual, such as varying financial income, different accommodation issues and severity of the disability. These discrepancies are allowed for by discussing a number of different solutions to problems in each case, whereas my autobiography concentrated chiefly on my own experiences at university and how I dealt with them. Third, there will also be a number of new topics reviewed, some which are not discussed at all in my first publication, such as an episode about the uncertainty of plumbers. The book takes the approach that having a positive mental attitude, and having the ability to break problems down into smaller constructive achievable tasks first, is fundamental in enabling one to make progress in life.

Chapter 2, 'An Overview of Autism', gives an overall introduction to the characteristics of the topic, and comments on the bewildering array of different symptoms that can occur with separate individuals with autism/Asperger's. It considers a number of issues, including the importance of getting the right diagnosis and professional help as early as possible, the vital role of social services after educational support ceases, and financial issues and concerns for parents and families.

Chapter 3, 'The Worry of the "What If?" Scenario', investigates how we autistic people can often build things up in our minds and become convinced that we are in danger or that something terrible might happen to us, long before anything actually does threaten us. Quite often there could be a sequence of events where the occurrence of one would imply the happening of a second event, and this in turn imply a third, and so on, which ultimately could lead to the final event, which would be the root cause of concern for the individual. For instance, event 1 – forgot to turn bath taps off; event 2 – flood in house implying event 3 – no cloths to clean up flood implying event 4 – the real concern being left homeless as house not safe to live in with dangerous electrics in the damp. A number of examples are given.

Chapter 4, 'The Vital Role of Communication', is a discussion on the absolute necessity for autistic youngsters to be able to communicate effectively and confidently with parents, teachers and mentors, in terms of both sending and receiving information. The chapter points out the fact that there are plenty of alternative methods of exchanging dialogue in addition to verbal speech alone, not always a practical option, and gives an illustration in some detail of a number of these forms of assistance. These include sign language, computer aids and physical activities. The importance of precise instruction is emphasised, and a humorous example of what can happen when this is not given is offered.

Chapter 5, 'The Art of Independent Living', offers some first-hand tips and pieces of advice on how to make the challenges of everyday independent living a little easier, and less daunting. It is particularly suitable for those who have recently moved into their own accommodation for the first time, with only minimum support from care workers and social services. The initial stress of moving house in the first place can be one of the most challenging experiences in anyone's life, but we see here that with careful planning and a strategy for prioritising situations as they arise, it is possible to cope much better in dealing with them and not be overwhelmed. Methods discussed include the use of written solutions to anxieties, the use of the telephone and the use of a 'record book' that is kept in the house. There is a discussion on the organisation and handling of food and money, advice on housework and suggestions about using public transport to and from home, together with an illustration of the importance of generalising a situation and being adaptable, with an example of what can happen otherwise.

Chapter 6, 'Rules of Socialising', is a chapter that I would not have been able to write as well just two years ago, since it is only recently I have experienced more of the socialising world. Making friends is exactly what we find difficult, and represents a mind-boggling array of different rules that seem to be different in each case. This chapter attempts to break down some of the challenges involved, by offering a number of general points of advice that can be followed in most situations. Key points covered are the importance of not doing too much or being too ambitious to begin with, arrangements for meetings and travel, good dress sense, financial considerations and respecting people's boundaries. A number of different locations are included, from shopping centres and cinemas to day trips and holidays. I also discuss here in some detail advice on trying new foods for the first time, having attempted it myself after a lifetime of a very restricted diet, and emphasise the fact that this was helpful not only in terms of being more healthy for my own point of view, but also in 'fitting in' better and not appearing unusual in a given situation where others were all eating different items.

Chapter 7, 'Further Education and Training Survival Guide', gives a comprehensive guide to the key aspects of life for the ambitious autistic hopeful, from advice on gaining a place in your chosen subject area and getting on the right course, to financial implications and accommodation issues. It is important that all staff working with parents and social services understand the condition and provide sympathetic support when appropriate. A concise and rigid timetable is not always provided at university or college, and great care must be taken to ensure an adequate strategy to manage workloads. It will often be the little things such as social issues or minor practical tasks and oral exams that prove the more challenging things for the autistic person. Some examples are given of the sort of traps and difficulties one can fall into, and suggestions on how one might deal with them are provided.

Chapter 8, 'The World of Sport as an Aid', explains how productive it can be for an autistic person to become involved in a sport, not only for feelings of achievement and self-worth, but also for the learning process in relating to others. A number of aspects are considered, from physical considerations and correct outfit, to the mental approaches and challenges of sport, to the value of sportsmanship and etiquette of players, and the importance of having a game plan and an understanding of the unspoken rules of a game. The chapter also touches on the art of giving sport coaching to others, using the example of a local sports club.

Chapter 9, 'The Challenge of Sharing Ideas with the Wider Audience', is about becoming a confident presenter, which can be an art in itself, as it is important not just to know your subject but to be able to communicate it effectively and in such a manner as to keep your audience interested. This chapter explores the tips of the trade and some of the do's and don'ts of giving local and public presentations, including how to calm nerves, the importance of overall design and back-up plans, and how to deal with answering difficult questions from the audience. Also included are sections on preparing work for publication, from small articles to entire books. There is in addition some advice about appearing on TV for those lucky enough to get the opportunity. There is never any excuse for allowing a disability to stop us performing in front of others, and one can always use some of the alternative forms of interaction with others from Chapter 4, if these prove necessary. This is the positive, bold approach of Chapter 9.

Chapter 10, 'Dealing with Uncertainty', begins with a detailed instance in my own life where I had to come to terms with a situation involving a lot of uncertainties, involving a group of plumbers and some defective items in my house. It then generalises the situation and asks how, in retrospect, another individual could have developed ways of putting certain plans into action and to cope with something similar happening to them. The chapter emphasises the fact that there are some things which are beyond our control, but there is no reason why we cannot adapt and use our known resources and skills to deal with a situation in a professional manner.

Chapter 11, 'Autism in a Nutshell', reviews the progress that has been made so far in autism awareness and aid by various places of authority such as schools, universities and social service departments, and suggests what the key targets such places should be attempting to set and achieve in the next few years in order to continue this. In many cases the physical requirements are available but the finances and mental will are not, and this chapter emphasises the importance of different groups (such as education, social services and parents) working in unison to enable major breakthroughs to occur and be recorded. It also suggests ways of ensuring that communication is good enough between the various groups to avoid mishap and individuals slipping though the net, so to speak, and ending up with inappropriate help (or no help at all!).

Appendix 1, 'Fun with Numbers!', is very different. It is very common for autistic individuals to be very gifted in one particular area of the sciences, the art world or music, having an eye for detail. In my own case it is the love of mathematics, and the often precise nature of the subject can appeal to many of us who like things to be orderly and exact. This appendix attempts to give an insight into some of my (and no doubt countless other people's) interest in the subject and shows, in particular, how apparently simple problems at first appearance can become more and more complicated. The important parallel comparison to this is that there will often be simple practical tasks, such as putting a shirt and tie on properly and folding the collar down in the right way, which can become almost unassailable tasks if not given appropriate help. But do not worry, I am not expecting everyone to understand all of the maths here!

CHAPTER 2

An Overview of Autism

2.1 Exactly what is autism?

Despite much progress in the field in recent years, the term 'autism' is still misunderstood, unheard of or even feared by many people who may feel uncomfortable or embarrassed about being in our company, arguing that our behaviour is often hard to grasp. In my lifetime as a man with autism, I have often been asked to sum up the properties of the condition in a couple of sentences, but this can be surprisingly difficult, as there is an enormous range of different kinds of autism and severities of it within each of those types, and what helps one of us may not help another. Autism is a complex disorder that affects our social and communicational development, and thus can be much harder for outsiders to spot than a more obvious disability such as a person bound to a wheelchair. This difficulty of recognition can be especially apparent to those of you who lie at the higher-functioning end of the autistic spectrum (which includes Asperger's Syndrome). Often to others you will appear virtually like any other confident person for much of the time, perhaps making friends or forming relationships, only to be left vulnerable to heartbreak or be taken advantage of simply because others failed to grasp the full symptoms of our disability or have used it as an excuse to exploit our weaknesses. You may feel intense frustration set in when trying to understand the rules and etiquette of successful socialising. These, which can appear to change with every situation you are in, can seem as overwhelming to us as it can be for a non-autistic person to grasp our own bewildering range of autistic behavioural patterns.

Autism is often associated with us having a learning disability in a more general sense (i.e. not merely a difficulty in social development but including other factors of impairment such as epilepsy, dyslexia and cerebral palsy) but this is not always the case, with the more able among us in particular appearing to have no obvious difficulty in learning. However, there is a certain number of characteristics that tend to occur in all cases of our condition. These include difficulties in reading social messages, taking things literally and being unable to tell the difference between fact and fiction or forms of sarcasm (we shall be examining such cases in a little more detail later in the book). These misunderstandings can lead us to perform inappropriate behaviour in the eyes of others, and to emotional problems. Remember that it is not just the words used by someone else that can cause difficulty (such as 'Go and wash your hands in the toilet' – make sure you wash them in the basin, *not* physically in the toilet itself!); many of us have an inability to recognise different facial expressions to tell if someone is happy or sad, or to sum up an individual by the manner of their dress sense or leisure-time activities. It may be very tempting for you to talk for hours about your special hobby. Indeed I have to admit my guilt on discussing aspects of higher mathematics for ages to almost anyone when I was younger, simply because I enjoyed it, so assumed they would as well. This is not, however, an assumption that can always be made. We risk interrupting or introducing topics at inappropriate times and others remarking on our lack of imagination in a social sense if we proceed in this reckless manner. For example, not everyone is interested in trying to solve a tenth-degree polynomial equation!

2.2 How can I tell others about the effects of my disability?

One of the chief difficulties for others trying to understand what life is like for you being autistic is the fact that most of them are simply not experiencing it themselves, and so in order to make progress it is often a good idea if we can make some parallel comparisons to autism's effects by trying to relate it to happenings and events that may occur in their everyday lives and that they will understand. To illustrate the type of things I have in mind, let us examine some examples that I have used to explain to others how our minds can operate.

2.2a *The degree of despair we can reach over apparently trivial situations*

This example centres on the fact that many autistic individuals are susceptible to loud sounds! Once you have your listener's undivided attention, you could state the following: 'Let us picture a situation where we have two red sports cars, identical in design, but one is a matchbox toy, the other the real thing. An autistic person is present inside the room where the toy lies, on top of a wooden table, with a hard floor of exposed floorboards below the table. Now let us consider the real car: its occupant is sitting inside with the vehicle parked on the side of a road next to a bridge which runs over a motorway below. We now suppose that two events suddenly occur, one to each individual discussed, and consider their feelings. Suppose that you went into the room with the autistic person and slid the toy car across the top of the table so that it was no longer centralised, but precariously balanced on the very edge of the table so it might fall off at any minute. And if it did so, it would make a loud clatter on the floor below. What now if you left the room again? The autistic person has noticed the car and becomes terribly aware of the possibility of it falling and making a noise. He is extremely disturbed by this and must remove the source of danger. He races across the room. But he cannot reach the car! The table is too high. A feeling of utter hopelessness is formed. A dread so great that words have difficulty describing it.'

Make sure at this point that your listener is still paying attention, then continue! 'Let us consider the event that occurs to our other person in the full-sized car. There has been a sudden earthquake. The car is shaken about by a landslide on the bridge close to where it is parked. Suddenly the car is sliding. It comes to a halt with two wheels hanging over the bridge. There is a creak and a groan. The whole structure could collapse in a few minutes. If it does so, the vehicle will crash onto the motorway. The traffic on the motorway has started moving again speedily after the tremors. The consequences of falling could be unthinkable. The occupant desperately tries to get out of the vehicle, and cannot! The doors have been damaged and will not open. Then the car starts sliding again. Any further movement on the driver's part will mean falling off the bridge. He must sit motionless and hope someone else will rescue him. His feeling of dread and hopelessness is total. Now the interesting fact of this comparison is that both our autistic individual and our driver are currently experiencing the *same level* of emotion with their apparent predicament. *Exactly* identical intensities of fear and stress, and of not being in control of the situation. This fact might be hard to grasp, but it is true for some of us autistic people!'

Having said so much, it is important to also include a possible happier ending scenario to your listener, to illustrate how obtaining the right sort of help can make all the difference for autistic people. You could perhaps continue: 'Suppose you now go back into the room with the table and push the toy car gently, so it once again rests comfortably on top and away from the edges. Suppose also that an emergency pick-up truck suddenly notices our driver's plight, and just in time hooks on to the vehicle and pulls it to safety before freeing our trapped individual. The intensity of relief and sensation of being safe again is clear to see on the autistic person's face. His heart will no longer pound. His body will no longer shake with anxiety. And his feelings on the matter will be every bit as great as our driver knowing that he is now out of danger after seemingly facing death at close quarters. So next time your autistic son or daughter, or the autistic person that you know, tells you something that appears to be totally trivial, it is worth considering this life/death comparison. Not all of us autistic individuals are quite as acutely affected as this. With the correct methods of treatment, much can be done to reduce anxiety levels. But such anxiety does exist, and is something we should be aware of.'

2.2b Feelings of incredible isolation

Here you could explain to your listener that feeling isolated is a state that some of us can be in almost continuously throughout our lifetime, and this is not just related to feeling different, but also because of missed opportunities. You could now phrase the following: 'Let us return once more to our imagined car (the real-sized one) and picture another scene where you have just seen your long-lost friend from the United States, whom you have not seen for five years, inside it. The car is sitting at traffic lights as you spot it, and you start to run towards it. Reaching out your arm, you can almost touch it, but suddenly in the last two seconds before your reach the car, the lights change and it speeds off. Despite calling out your friend's name and waving at them, they did not even see you. And you do not have their telephone number so you cannot contact them later. You think: "If only I had been a couple of seconds earlier! If only I had reacted differently, or gone to the other side of the car they probably would have seen me. It is so frustrating!" In a parallel sense the autistic person's mind is full of thoughts such as "If only I could have spoken to that nice-looking girl" or "If only I had made friends with just one of my school class by saying the right thing instead of putting everyone off by telling everyone facts that bored them all, like there are 257 houses between my house and the school, and 203 fences between them!" Or alternatively picture a scene where you can only watch the rest of the pupils play games from a distance and never join in. If we form a vision of these feelings of isolation and frustration all the time instead of isolated moments in your life, we can conjure up the state that those with our disability can be in for years on end if they remain without appropriate assistance.'

2.2c *What about recognising other symptoms of autism?*

I have usually given the following account through my own experiences when asked this question (you can of course invent your own examples depending your circumstances, so long as they are clear and your listener understands them). 'Lack of social interaction is not the only recognisable characteristic of autism. There are many other possible clues: spinning objects repeatedly, lack of eye contact, talking in a robotic manner or in parrot fashion. There is often a total lack among us of the so-called "inquisitive questions" that most young children go through (in asking their parents things) to develop their learning process about the world. In addition, we may perform bizarre rituals such as rotating our bodies, swinging our arms and legs around, or making strange sounds and laughing excessively for no apparent reason to the outsider. Some of these actions may be used as a way of protection from the rest of the world. I used to pretend to be a robot who was unaffected by youngsters who teased me, as it helped me to release my frustration about being bullied. Sometimes it may be because some worry or anxiety has been built up out of all proportion in our mind through feeling trapped by a situation, having been unable to discuss it properly with others. While this sort of behaviour can be upsetting, our parents should bear in mind that it is often better that we use the actions to indicate a problem rather than not communicating to them and suffering in silence, in which case the difficulty may never be discovered.'

2.3 What do I tell my parents if they are at a loss as to how to help me?

If you have not already been formally diagnosed with autism, your parents or carers should be approaching a local diagnostic team specifically trained in the condition, a referral to which is normally made by your local doctor (if no such referral is made, parents or carers – or you – should contact the National Autistic Society directly). Any other type of team assigned to help you just will not do, as people without the proper know-how could make matters worse for you rather than better, just like a builder constructing a house without firm foundations. If we do not get our basics right, then any apparent form of progress that we have built up could come tumbling down at any moment. So if your parents are not doing this, you need to ask them to! You may have to work quite hard at this as well, because getting this right form of help is often harder than it looks. Parents often encounter difficulties when no such aid is available in the county that you live in, and they may not be given any financial support if they try to let you attend a school in another county. However, the importance of proper aid can never be underestimated. Take it from me, if I had not received this specialist help when I was younger, I have no doubt I would not be writing this book in my independently run home today, but would probably be stuck inside a mental institution somewhere with no future prospects whatsoever of making progress, simply because others did not believe in my ability. To deny any person the right to maximum achievement is an utter sin that should not be allowed.

2.4 The power of persuasion

You may need to call on your initiative when requesting that you require the correct help to improve your standard of life and well-being. Some parents may not like the idea of you being labelled with a disability such as autism in the first place. They may feel vaguely guilty and believe that in some way it could be their fault that you have not developed properly in a social sense. They could fear prejudice from other people, and wonder how those others might react. However, the first step in solving a problem is to define formally what that problem is, and your parents must realise that in the long run they are doing you a favour by getting you a diagnosis as soon as possible (it can be done as early as two years old). So tell your parents how much worse it might be if you become a teenager or young adult having made virtually no progress either academically or socially and have become very withdrawn, simply because you did not receive the proper care. If they are still not convinced, you may have to resort to some more of our parallel examples, for instance:

> *Example 1*: You could state 'Imagine a long distance snow trekker walking to the North Pole – he could not afford to ignore a developing hole in his boots, but should replace them, to avoid the situation deteriorating with every step until he is almost walking barefoot. It may be too late to save himself by that time.'

> *Example 2*: Quote 'Consider a person who had been given the opportunity of a far better type of lifestyle, more qualifications, a better job and improved social life if he moves house once to the next county. Clearly the man would be very likely to put up with the temporary inconvenience of moving, knowing that his longer-term prosperity is in the balance.'

Similarly, your parents should realise that if moving house is required to get you into an area with appropriate help then it is usually better to move!

2.5 Outside help for your parents

Do not be surprised if your parents sometimes end up feeling lonely, frustrated or even angry at times upon your diagnosis. Remember that they have feelings as well as you, and there are times that they need help. They often find considerable comfort in being able to talk to other parents in a similar situation. This is possible for them through parent evenings at schools and colleges, and also autistic conferences. The National Autistic Society has details of (and even organises) many of these events, and I know through my own experience of performing talks as a public lecturer that even one such visit can have an extremely reassuring effect. On one occasion, one particular lady burst into tears upon hearing me talking, and my first impression was 'Oh dear, whatever is the matter?' In fact these tears were those of intense relief that she was at last able to relate to someone who had displayed similar symptoms to that of her own autistic youngster, having spent many years being unable to do so. She also learnt (through me) that it is possible for autistic individuals like us to make progress, achieve goals and run almost completely independent lives. I have always said that your parents should trust their instincts about suspecting you have the condition and not listen to the inexperienced people (and you should not either!) who do not know what they are talking about. One doctor, for example, once told me when I was about six years old that I was mentally retarded and beyond hope of any improvement. Well I am now a fully fledged author with two maths degrees... In addition, once you are diagnosed and arrangements have been made to begin the correct trained support, your parents will then have the extra satisfaction and reassurance of observing the times when you do start making more progress than before.

2.6 Do not run before you can walk

Both your parents and you must realise that there are occasions when you must not be too hard on yourselves. None of you can expect miracles straight away just because specialised help has started, nor a sudden and immediate transformation of your ability to cope with every new situation after a life full of trauma and anxiety. Instead we should be prepared to allow time before noticing significant advancements. Your parents should not blame themselves for a situation beyond their control. This is one of the reasons why seeking out professional help in the first place is so crucial in helping us share the load of caring. For certain individuals, some form of respite care may be appropriate. This can provide vital experience for you in the learning process of interacting with other people, although you may not like this idea at first! As a youngster, there was a time when I started spending some periods away from my parents' home, in a hostel for young people with disabilities, to learn more about independence. At first this was just for a few hours a day, but was gradually built up into me spending the week there and going back to my parents at the weekend. At the time my mother was becoming ill with cancer and it was an immense relief for her to have these rest periods where she did not have to worry about my well-being. This point is in fact generally true for parents in that although respite care may seem a soft option or a guilty one in their minds, it can give them a vital gap from the constant stress of bringing up their children. (It is amazing how much difference even a short break can make to them feeling more refreshed and ready to start again.) Moreover, although I may not have been keen at the time, the experience I gained there played a crucial part in the foundation of my independent life today.

2.7 Help for you from social services later in life

It is almost certain that you will continue to need assistance at least in some form after leaving mainstream schooling. Social services aim to bridge the sudden absence of assistance that would otherwise result in this change of circumstances, and provide help to ensure your continued development and well-being. This help can be given in various forms, from day centres and full-time special needs homes to occasional visits from trained staff, and can give aid to aspects of employment, finance and organising social events, for instance. If you are staying in a care home, you will often be able to use the staff present to help you go out to places where you can meet others. These could include events such as local sports fixtures, a meal in a pub or restaurant, or going to the gym, the cinema or theatre, for example. Equally they could provide help in accompanying you to an interview for an important job, with advice on how to go about it. The type and amount of help you will receive will depend partly on your individual situation and how much progress in independence you have already made. It is worth remarking that we should have the same legal rights as others in the population, so that anyone discriminating against you, such as offering you a reduced level of service (or even refusing service altogether), is doing so illegally and can be taken to court. Your local council should have a written policy on their methods of helping people with disabilities and the sort of services they provide, so you may be interested to read it to verify that they are indeed sticking to their word.

2.8 Be positive but realistic with goals

For you, as an autistic individual, there may often be times in your life when it can be easier to accept things as they are, especially in terms of happenings that are beyond your control. You should not always dwell too much on your difficulties (although it is a good idea to work on them) but be positive about what you are good at, and make an effort to get even better. For instance, I try not to get too depressed about the fact that I shall probably never marry or have a serious relationship because of my social vulnerability, but instead take comfort from the fact that I am giving talks on autism across the country and working hard to improve the lives of thousands of other families through my experiences. The satisfaction of being able to help so many others more than makes up for the things I have found harder to do. Every day can be part of the learning curve, and only the other day one student asked me what I thought was an extremely intelligent question: 'In view of the recent scientific controversy about whether there is a definite link between the MMR vaccine and autism, what is your personal view, as someone with autism, on the matter?' But I was unable to give a precise answer. What mattered here was that I was honest, remarking that perhaps no one yet knows for certain, as there is not enough hard evidence (a debatable point of view!) and that I was not sure. Honesty and trust are two of the fundamental foundations on which we can build friendships and respect from others which can enrich and bring happiness and contentment into our lives, in whatever form that may take.

CHAPTER 3

The Worry of the 'What If?' Scenario

3.1 Anxieties often arise because of happenings in your past

In this chapter I shall be describing how the mind of the autistic individual can produce worries which, if not dealt with properly, can escalate out of all proportion. The night-time in particular can be a breeding ground for many anxieties, as the mind is often free to wander. In my bedroom, when I was young, only part of the floor was covered with carpet, the remaining area (near to my bed) being left as a set of exposed floorboards. I used to look closely at these boards, sometimes for what seemed like hours at a time, staring in particular at the various 'knotted' darker areas. I used to imagine that these knots represented people who were 'stuck' in the surrounding lighter areas, which were likened to quicksand. Of course, the knots never moved, so it was as if these imaginary people were stuck there for ever, with a feeling of hopelessness. Perhaps I was relating this to my own predicament, being autistic and feeling totally different, but often trapped with isolation, an isolation that never seemed to go away; although at this time I had not been formally diagnosed.

3.2 The majority of anxieties can be resolved

One critical observation is the fact that as much as 99 per cent of the things that worried me never actually happened. Autistic people can waste an incredible amount of energy getting every part of their body tensed up in a state of anxiety while dwelling on something that they will probably never have to face. What if one of us had a dentist appointment a week on Thursday, but then wished to catch a bus half an hour later to see a friend? The list of possible worries is endless. What if you get delayed at the dentist and as a result miss the bus to the friend? What if you cannot get through to this friend on the telephone to let her know you missed the bus, as there is no telephone box nearby? What if your friend is cross with you, thinking you have missed seeing her on purpose? It is so easy to get sucked into a 'worry mode' when your whole body can feel heavy and ache all over. I once pulled a muscle after a whole week of feeling tense in this way. And then took another week to recover. At least when one is so engrossed in one worry, it might stop others at the time.

More often than not, all the anxiety turns out to be for nothing. Thursday week arrives, you are longer than usual at the dentist and the bus to your friend left five minutes late anyway, so you need not have rushed to the bus station. You may then think to yourself, 'What a fool! All that worry for nothing!' Then there might be a couple of hours of tranquillity with no major anxieties in your mind. This can feel truly wonderful; all your muscles can relax. Then, horror of horrors, something else happens to start the alarm bells ringing for 'worry mode'. And so it goes on. The worries that you had forgotten about, such as dirty marks on the toothpaste tube or a broken toy, have now resurfaced because you sorted out the initial worries. How can we stop this never-ending cycle making us a nervous wreck? The thing is to *do* something about it. The actual process of worry and anxiety will never physically or practically help us. Taking simple, real actions to prevent the worries coming true will help.

3.3 Oversleeping

3.3a The fear of oversleeping

I used to be paranoid about the risk of oversleeping. Anything important early the next morning such as a school exam, or interview, or trip involving an early bus or train had me in such a state of anxiety I would often wake up hours earlier, say 4 or 5 a.m. I would be more anxious about this than the activity itself. And often when I was more relaxed (such as at the weekend) I would wake up later, so it was as if I could not let myself relax when I did have to get up early, since I knew I should wake up early anyway if I was tense. But this was an exhausting way of making sure I was awake on time. I used to make my mum or dad promise to make sure I was up in time when I needed to be. But even then I panicked. I tried to doubt my own memory. Half an hour after they promised, I would think, 'Did I definitely tell them the right time, and the correct date?' Often, as a youngster, I would wake my parents up several times in the middle of the night for constant reassurance on this, that they would not forget to wake me. There could be many readers out there who can relate to similar experiences, so how does one develop a strategy for dealing with them?

3.3b How to deal with the oversleeping anxiety

Practically, the logical step to ensuring one does not oversleep is to buy an alarm clock. Simple? Perhaps for some. But not for many autistic people. That is not the end of the story! If the alarm clock is powered from the mains, what if there is a power cut and it does not go off? You could still oversleep. If it is battery operated, what if the batteries run down in the middle of the night, so that it fails to work either? Even if there is no power cut or battery failure, have you definitely set the alarm for the correct time, and switched it on properly? Some of us might end up checking these details on our alarms five or six times a night. What if you suddenly notice a layer of dust lying all over the clock? Will that affect the alarm working? Should you then reset the alarm to go off now, just to make sure it still rings? And then there is the alternative worry that you might set the alarm by mistake at a time when you do not need to get up and be woken up unnecessarily. How do we find our way through this minefield of potential worries that most people may not even think about very much?

My current solution for waking-up assurance is the ownership of two alarm clocks; one timed to go off two minutes after the other to allow for snoozing time. They are both battery operated to avoid the risk of a power cut. I check the batteries regularly to ensure they are fresh enough to operate and not running low on energy. Even if one of the alarm clocks suddenly malfunctioned, the chances of the other one doing the same are too small to concern me. The clocks are of a simple design, with instructions that can be clearly understood, so I am absolutely sure when I have set the alarms and for what time. I dust the clocks regularly to avoid dust settling on them in any great quantity. I can also tell straight away when the alarm is in the off position, for weekends or holiday times. Although we can never foresee every possible occurrence, we can certainly devise a system such as this, which eliminates all the major worries and reduces stress to a minimum.

3.4 Worries founded on past events

Another factor that might set off an obsession or worry might be a certain pattern of sounds that could be related to something else, perhaps that worried you in the past, or that would make you feel vulnerable. When, as a youngster, I put my head against the pillow on my bed I used to hear the blood pulsing in my ear. This sounded like the footsteps of someone or something large walking through tall grass. I used to imagine that this was a monster who was gradually getting closer and closer to me with every step. Sometimes I would then lift my head off the pillow so that the footsteps would stop. Usually this would help, but if I was especially anxious I then imagined that the footsteps had stopped because the monster had reached me and would devour me any second. I even jumped out of bed screaming on occasions. Having already been chased or followed around the school playground by bullies who said they were going to 'get me', perhaps I had that fear subconsciously in my mind when thinking about the imagined monster.

3.5 More about worries founded on past events

3.5a Dog fears

There are some anxieties or fears that autistic people have that are due to an obvious cause such as an occurrence earlier in life. These events can stay with you for years in graphic detail. I personally have a great fear of dogs, having been attacked and bitten on several occasions. Two of these stand out. One year, round about fireworks night, our family had decided to go to one of the organised displays, but the place was difficult to find in the dark and by mistake we attempted to gain entrance to the field through the wrong gate. Unknown to us, a guard dog was about, trained to attack intruders. He went straight for me and I ended up in hospital for an injection to prevent developing a disease. Another time, I was walking home from work when an enormous German shepherd dog jumped over the fence of a nearby house just as its family had arrived home, and despite me walking on trying to take no notice, the animal swiftly grabbed hold of my leg and would not let go until I screamed. Perhaps I sweated more or my heart beat faster, but a dog will somehow always sense when you are afraid. And you knowing that the dog knows that will always make it worse.

3.5b Farm animal fears

My fear of animals was not restricted to dogs, but extended to other animals too. I was once made to ride a horse against my wishes in order to fit in with the group outing I was attending at the time. The other people did not want me to use my autism as an excuse not to ride. But I was petrified at the thought of being on another creature that I felt I could not control and had a mind of its own. I was concentrating so much on simply keeping my balance that I failed to notice a low overhanging tree along the track we were riding. I knocked straight into the branches, lost my grip and fell right off the horse, being lucky to escape it treading on me as I lay on the pathway. Later that day they made me get on the horse again, but I still sensed the animal knew I was uncomfortable, even though I did not fall off again. It was the same with farm animals such as cows and bulls. I always imagined the worst-case scenario when on a country walk, like a bull charging me, and even the animals eyeing me made me nervous. The bottom line is that there is that element of uncertainty and unpredictability about what these animals might do, or how they might behave, which I found frightening. Whenever possible, autistic individuals like to have things exact and to know what is going to happen, and life just is not like that most of the time.

3.5c Bee fears

Even animals of the smaller kind can be guilty of causing stress to the autistic individual. On one fairly innocent day of those long-forgotten days of childhood that seemed to last for ever, I happened to be exploring round the corners of the school playground when I suddenly noticed a shed-like construction with a small gap behind this and the border hedge. Being curious, I stepped a few feet into this gap, thinking maybe I could squeeze through and come out the other side of the shed. Suddenly I became aware of a noise, a constant humming noise that seemed very intense. Could it be an electrical generator, I thought? I knew these could sometimes make such noises. Then I turned my head slightly. And saw the movement. Bees! Thousands of them! The entire wall of the back of the shed was covered with them! They say that often stressful situations can be overwhelming to autistic people. But when you (or any other human being) are in a situation where you must help yourself, your own protective system comes into play. You just act on instinct, even when you may be frozen with fear.

3.5d Escape the danger!

My first thought was, 'I've got to get out of here'. Not quickly. I had seen horror movies when people had panicked and been smothered by the insects. 'I must keep calm', I kept thinking, 'I must keep calm'. Slowly I stepped backwards away from the persistent humming. Back in the open! Freedom. I thought I had escaped. 'I don't believe that just happened, but it's over now', I thought, as I walked back across the playground towards the school. Then I felt the pain of a sting. Well, I was bound to get one sting. But then another, and another. Suddenly I am running through the school corridors screaming! Some of the bees had got under my clothes. It took several adults to get rid of them and calm me down. But by the time they had done so, I had about eight or nine stings. I recovered physically in about a week, but mentally I shall never forget this incident. When every anxiety of an individual's life can be heightened by autism, one tends to remember those anxieties vividly, even years later. These memories can manifest themselves in unusual behaviour from us.

3.5e Facing your animal fears

I do not like insects – full stop. Even today, if I see a wasp or bee in a restaurant flying even remotely near my table, I would rather go to the other side of the room, always assuming the worst. If I see one on a bus when I am on it, I shall be compelled to watch it through the whole journey for fear of a sting. Even if I am talking to someone, I have to carry on looking at the insect, perhaps for an hour or two if that is how long my journey will take. If I knew the buses ran regularly, I might even get off this one at the next bus stop and catch the next one just to have a stress-free journey. Recently I have started going round to some friends who have dogs and have also persuaded me not to be too paranoid about the

insects. It is usually best to face your fears, even if only in modera-
tion at first. Just being close to both types of creature has reassured
me that they are not all bad, and that I am still here to tell the tale.
If we never take any risks, we may be safe, but like a bird stuck in a
cage, where can we go and what progress can we make? Being
brave can set us free from that imprisonment to a new life of independence – yes, there will be challenges and things may not
always go our way, but when they do we can achieve goals to
make ourselves proud.

3.6 The worry chain

3.6a The worry-chain formation

There are some worries that autistic people have which involve
the fear of one event leading to another, with the second happening leading to a third and fourth and so on. Such anxieties can
often result from a change of circumstances or responsibility.
When I was a child, one of my biggest fears was of somehow
getting lost or isolated from my parents, and feeling in a state of
hopelessness about how to cope. After all, whenever I was with
my parents they would always make sure I was safe, not only at
home but in shops too, where they would always sort out the
matter of paying the bill in a restaurant or treating me to a new
toy. However, there came a time when I had to learn to take
responsibility for handling money. I was, even at an early age, very
good with figures, and it did not take me long to recognise most
currency and how to use it. But as so often in the past, that autistic
mind feverishly looking for anxieties now managed to build a
concern for an event that could lead to a second event and then a
third (the 'what if?' scenario phobia), this concern building up out
of all proportions. Let us examine these possible events.

3.6b An example of a worry-chain formation

My mind operated as follows. Nobody is perfect. Suppose I went
into a shop and forgot to pay by mistake – or suppose I did pay,

but incorrectly. This would be the first event. I had heard some horror stories about people who were taken to court when they had forgotten to pay for something like a few cabbages. So suppose, as a result of this first event, the shop owner then reported me to the authorities, resulting in a set of policemen tracking me down at my house hours later that day. These men of authority would then force me into their car and drive me straight to the nearest prison and lock me in there. As a result of this a third event would occur, which was the underlying fear of the whole situation in the first place, namely that I would be stuck in a place away from my parents, feeling I had no control over what happened to me next. Not one of these things ever happened in real life, yet the fear of the possibility that they might do seemed real enough to me at the time. It took constant reassurance and several months of convincing before I would even step in a shop again, and I soon found that going in a shop with other people made the whole prospect even more frightening than taking the chance on my own.

Things had been simple when my parents had paid for everything and at least when I was on my own I knew I had to pay. But now, suppose I went in with a friend or a relative? No one had told me who pays for things in that case, and it seemed to be different almost every time when watching other people I knew. What if I assumed I had to pay for everything, and my friend had already paid for me? Or worse, what if I had assumed my friend would pay for everything like my parents used to, and they had not, resulting in neither of us coughing up the cash? I had no concept then of the fact that the norm is for everyone to pay for themselves, unless specifically stated otherwise. Even when other people had assured me that we had paid, I would still have to remember it. It is perhaps not so bad in, say, a restaurant, where you pay as you go out, and it is fresh in your mind. But in other places you pay first. You could then spend half an hour having a coffee, discussing other things with your mind wandering, and then suddenly when it is time to leave the premises you could think, 'Did I pay? Can I trust my memory of this?' I have done this on numerous occasions, but then developed strategies to deal with them.

3.6c How the worry chain can affect you

I can vividly remember occasions when my phobias over payment made me react to people in ways which were almost against my wishes. On one occasion a friend had kindly offered to give me a lift home in her car, but when about two-thirds of the way home she asked me if we could go to a local garage for a few minutes for her to fill up on fuel before taking me the rest of the way home, as she was getting very low on petrol and was concerned that she would not have enough to get herself home otherwise. I insisted, however, that I was in a great hurry and really wanted to go home immediately. She was rather flustered at this, and could not understand why I was in such a worried state and panic to get home, where a few minutes before I was perfectly relaxed. The real reason for me wishing to avoid the garage is that no one had told me who would in fact pay for the petrol there. True, it was her car, but I was in it as well! Then I would be vulnerable to the same fear as in the shops. Worse still, I did not feel I could tell her this for fear of looking foolish because people like me were surely supposed to know such things.

3.6d How to break the chain

Initially I started taking a small notepad into shops and restaurants with me, and would tick off on the paper that I had 'paid in this place'. This significantly reduced anxiety, but it was also rather clumsy and could be regarded as only a short-term solution. The problem, ultimately, is that we have to blend in or fit in with society to a reasonable degree. And making notes on pads on whether we have paid in every single shop is not the norm. How many other people do you know who scribble away every time they buy a paper or a packet of crisps? By all means, use this system initially if it helps you to get going. But ultimately we have to learn to trust our own memories. We have to realise that if there is a query with payment and the person serving you is not satisfied, they will call you back and attempt to resolve it before you leave. We have to learn to trust our friends if they say they have paid, even if we cannot physically see them handing over any cash. They could have done this when we were not looking, or have paid with a card, when the money is automatically deducted from their bank account without directly touching any money, a way of paying that is becoming increasingly popular these days.

The important thing about this for other autistic people to note is that we must learn through experiences such as these, so that we are more able to handle a similar event next time it occurs. It is perhaps a good thing to make a note on paper, telling you who pays for petrol and at car parks. Once this is done it can be kept at home for future reference and whenever you find yourself doubting your memory, you can refer to these notes for reassurance. In my experience, as you gain more confidence in these things (and you have to face them to do that) you *will* start trusting your memory and the fact that at the end of the day it is *their* car (not yours), and they are responsible for buying fuel or a car-parking ticket. There are a few exceptions to this general rule, for example if your friend regularly gave you lifts each week you might offer them some money towards the petrol (it would be the decent thing to do), but even then they would normally still do the actual physical buying of the fuel and you would pay them back later, unless it has been specifically agreed otherwise.

3.7 Do I keep a secret?

Another trap that can be fallen into if one is not prepared is when to keep a secret, or a promise. Suppose, for instance, this child you know tells you one day that he has recently started smoking or perhaps even taking drugs. Then he tells you, 'Whatever you do, don't tell anyone – if my parents found out they'd go ballistic!'

This sort of remark can present a terrible dilemma for the autistic individual. On the one hand, if you keep your promise to this child because you have been asked to do so and took it literally, you may feel terribly worried about it and bottle things up, not feeling you can talk to anyone else to lighten the load, so to speak. On the other hand, if you do tell someone and ask their advice, then you have the worry of having broken the initial promise. Unfortunately the very act of getting closer to people in a normal social sense often involves sharing perhaps personal or confidential information with them that they probably will not want too many others to know about. It is often very hard for us to understand when and when not to tell others as it depends on individual circumstances.

It is often a good idea, if you are not certain about a particular situation, to consult a third (neutral) person and ask for advice (provided this is a tried and trusted friend or relative). You may be able to suss out the situation yourself by using common sense. For example, does the occurrence put anyone's health in peril? If your brother said to you, 'I've got Mum a brand new mobile for Christmas, she's got no idea, so don't say anything', there is no reason for telling anyone because no one would be in danger, and if you did, it would spoil the surprise. After all, would you like to know what all your Christmas presents were before you have opened them? On the other hand, if someone you know is taking drugs, there is a very real chance that they could end up causing themselves and their families grief, so in this case you usually would be justified in telling someone. Remember, you can always speak to a counsellor in the strictest confidence if the situation seems very complex or frightening and you feel you need help to sort it out. Numbers to contact these people are in the phone book and on the Internet.

3.8 Fear of items in your house

3.8a Fear of electricity

Even everyday household objects can create phobias that can build up enormously if unchecked. I used to have a constant fear of electric shocks to such an extent that I used to dream that my entire house was covered with cables all over the floors of each room. I used to have to tiptoe across the rooms in this dream without touching a single wire. If I did, I would immediately get a shock. This fear was probably a combination of hearing horror stories of people electrocuting themselves and the fact that, as an inexperienced child, I once tried to mend a broken computer by putting two live wires together – the blue sparks were flying! Although I escaped without a shock, the experience haunts me, yet another example of how events in earlier life can affect an individual years after. I also have a fear of a house fire, having watched one of those videos about how quickly one can spread through the house. The videos are a good idea for most people because they spur them on to take precautions such as fitting smoke alarms in the property, but in my case I became almost paranoid about the risk for a period, which even I now recognise was not reasonable.

3.8b Complications of minor details involving your house items

Making records of when things such as cookers and heaters are off or not, using descriptions and/or pictures on paper, is a good idea for reducing stress (see Chapter 5), but there are always additional factors that can complicate things. For example, you have a cooker where the 'off' indicator is that a pointer (mark on the knob) points directly at the number 0. However, suppose that this knob is slightly stiff and the marker does not point *exactly* to zero, although it is still very close to it. Are you then still safe or will the cooker be slowly building up heat without you realising it? Or suppose you went into someone else's kitchen, leaned down to pick up a dropped cookery book, and in doing so brushed gently against part of the kitchen work surface. Would it just have been the table top, or could you have accidentally pushed a switch to activate the washing machine which might result in your friend's kitchen getting flooded because they would not realise what had happened? Thoughts like these can run a seemingly never-ending cycle on occasions, so we must learn to control our anxieties before they spoil our enjoyment of life.

3.8c Overcoming phobias of house items

It is a good idea to know where the master (i.e. main wall) switch is to an appliance such as a cooker or washer. This provides an extra safety factor, in that so long as the mains power is not connected then the apparatus will not come on, even if the individual knobs are turned by mistake. Equally, it is good to know where the fuse box and water stopcock are in your property in case you do get a leaky water pipe or a power cut. If you are concerned about something in your friend's house, then by all means check with them to reassure you, but do not do so 18 times and spoil the whole day dwelling on it! Ultimately it is their house and their responsibility. In your own home, of course, you must be able to check these things. If you are uncertain about something, why not check with your support worker and make a note of it for future reference? And do not forget to keep this information in a safe place where you can find it easily. There is no point in writing down a hundred rules to reassure you about things, and then find you spend the whole evening looking for the notepad that you wrote it all in!

3.9 Worries can remain in your long-term memory

You may find memories of events that happened involving the actions of other people, perhaps that caused you worry, can sometimes spring back into your mind again after you have subconsciously forgotten them, while you were concentrating on more immediate concerns. My parents once bought me a hardback book when I was a young child, and I had noticed straight away that the last 'page' of this book appeared thicker than any of the others. I was convinced that this so-called single page was really two that were stuck together, but was not able to separate them. I showed several other people who after inspection, assured me (even promised absolutely in one case) that it definitely was only one page and that I was imagining the whole thing. I failed to be convinced though and, one day, when no one else was around, I pulled for ages on this part of the book, and sure enough, eventually it gave way, gradually, and piece by piece it came unstuck. It *was* two separate pages, and I felt a great surge of triumph, followed by a sense of annoyance that my usually so reliable mother had inadvertently misled me about it. Who knows, maybe being autistic heightens our awareness of certain things more than others, compensating for the fact that we can find it difficult to socialise, just like a blind man can develop an enhanced sense of his other four senses. I forget this 'book' event for ages and then sometimes it comes back to me again.

3.10 Intrusion into your world can be painful

Sometimes an intrusion can be an invasion of what in your mind is your private domain, rather than actual physical or verbal abuse, that can hurt. As a youngster, I used to love playing in a small wood just minutes' walk from my home. This wood was divided up into four main parts, and in each part a long line of trees stood where my sister, family and I used to try to climb across the branches of each tree in the line without putting our feet on the ground. Each part of the wood was such that it got progressively harder to do this, as the trees got more covered in ivy and other plants, and also stood further apart with fewer lower branches. We spent years having fun in the wood, playing games such as these until one day, in just a few hours, workmen from the local authorities cut down about half of our wood to make extra room on the adjoining playing field (for football matches). I was devastated looking at all the tree stumps and fallen branches – it was almost as if they had ripped away part of my childhood happiness in a place where I had felt safe and distant from the troubles of autistic life.

In conclusion, we realise through this chapter that there are many ways that a worry can develop among us and that other people are often unaware of the cause, which can make our lives all the more challenging. Finding a strategy to cope with these anxieties should be at the forefront of all autistic people's goals for living a more fulfilling life.

CHAPTER 4

The Vital Role of Communication

4.1 The essential necessities of dialogue

The ability of us autistic individuals to communicate effectively with human companions is fundamental to our development towards living a happy and successfully independent life. In order for dialogue to take place, we must be able to:

- receive information in an understandable form

- analyse the information and decide if a response is necessary

- send out a reply in a manner which is understandable and appropriate to the recipient.

In this chapter, we shall examine each of these necessities and the various forms they might take, and the possible problems and complications that might arise through an inability for some of us to carry out one or more of these criteria correctly.

As individuals we can receive information in many ways, speech and writing being the obvious, but also through sign and body language, computerised devices and the Internet, as well as telecommunications. Unfortunately things are not always so clear cut, because in certain situations other people around us often assume that we already have a number of supposed basic bits of knowledge, and thus these bits will not be explicitly stated to us. This type of occurrence can lead us into difficulties, particularly in social events (see Chapter 6) where our developmental skills in picking up rules of the norm can seem to our peers to be lagging behind. Unless our parents or carers are aware of our disability, this discrepancy may not be noticed until it is too late to avoid embarrassment. We now examine an example of just how awkward one can feel when experiencing this sort of predicament.

4.2 Consequences of the lack of precise instruction

As a young boy I was made (against my wishes) to participate in a game of football with the rest of my class. I had absolutely no interest in the game at the time, and no one had explicitly told me the basic rules of how to play. My only opportunity to collect data, it would seem, was by watching the other players kicking the ball around, since I had never managed to get anywhere near it myself. The only conclusion I could arrive at is that all the players had to try to get to the ball and then kick it as hard as they could and as far as they could. One day, and I really cannot remember how, I somehow ended up getting to the ball while everyone else was stuck in the opposite half of the playing field. 'Marc!' a voice shouted out from one of the players on my team who had spotted where I was, 'Go for it! Here's your chance to win us the game!' Well, I certainly did that, to the best of my knowledge. I kicked that ball like crazy, right to the edge of the field. And did I stop there? I did not! I continued on into the next field, then into the third one…and on and on for what seemed like miles! Oh sorry, I forgot about that small construction at the edge of the playing area, with two posts and a net they call a goal. No one had told me what *that* was for! Even the goalkeeper was down the other end of the field with the other players, and all I was supposed to do was kick the ball into this net once to win the game. It had been assumed that I knew this. But assumption was a rash thing for the others to make. Autistic people need precise instructions on all aspects of a game like this, even the things that people are expected to know automatically. After the game, I was as depressed as the rest of my team. While they asked, 'Marc, what on earth happened – you could have won us the game!' I was thinking, 'If only someone had *told* me the rules!'

4.3 When is participation more important than examination?

Another important point relating to us learning physical tasks for the first time, such as being able to dress properly, is to ensure that we do not merely watch our instructor carrying out the action, but attempt it ourselves. The process of putting one's tie on could be a good example here, because if you just watch someone else put their own tie on themselves (or even on you while they physically do the tying) it is quite likely that your memory of the process could go 'in one ear and out the other', so to speak. Usually only when you attempt to do your own tie up several times yourself can you get even remotely close to getting the hang of it effectively. Complications can sometimes arise when situations change slightly and we are unable or unprepared to make the necessary adjustments. Although I personally had been taught how to dress under a normal situation, I used to dread PE at school, as we were made to shower afterwards. This exposed my inability to dry myself thoroughly and consequently I struggled to get my clothes on again properly: it took a lot longer while my body was still wet. It ended up with me dreading this part more than the actual PE, as I was so conscious about the time and did not like being even one minute longer out of school. So try to look ahead and prepare beforehand if possible on how to deal with new challenges (ask your carer if necessary for help), once again making sure you attempt any physical learning process yourself.

4.4 An example of when we do not fit in

Some of you may have found yourselves having problems or feeling depressed as a result of having a playing activity or pastime that seems inappropriate to the rest of society, perhaps because you were not aware of this at the time through a lack of social exposure to others. For example, I used to have a go-kart which I persistently rode round my local estate, pretending to be a bus driver; this continuing until I was about 15 years old. One day I got considerably upset by another boy coming up to me and commenting, 'Aren't you a bit old to be riding around on that thing?' Although I understood what he was saying, and probably deep down knew that I was too old to do so and still appear normal, I would have much preferred to be left alone to carry on riding. After all, I was *enjoying* it. I was not capable then of confidently meeting friends or going out socialising. Now it was as if others wanted to deprive me of one of the few things I did enjoy. Ultimately, this boy possibly had my future welfare in mind and how I would be able to blend in with the rest of society, although I could not see it at the time.

Another time while I was riding along slowly and quietly round a cul-de-sac an elderly couple asked me to 'go away and never ride near there again', perhaps mistaking me for a yobbo! I certainly did not receive that information too happily, and was utterly bemused about what I had done wrong.

4.5 An example of when we can bottle feelings up

The ability to communicate effectively is important, not just in terms of the learning process but also for us to be able to express our concerns to others and discuss ways of dealing with them without bottling things up and becoming frustrated. If this ability is lacking, there may be a tendency for some of us to withdraw further into our own private world, and increase those activities that seem inappropriate to others. As a youngster I had a fixation with throwing inanimate objects: empty boxes down the stairs or wine gums along the pavements of roads. I would pretend that these items had become alive, and were a higher life form than humans, being able to escape the effects of any bullying or teasing that I myself was often subjected to. I would continue to look at the items only while they were still moving, since it was then much easier to visualise them as living. I was always aware, of course, deep down that these objects were not alive, but I had chosen this throwing habit simply as a way of getting rid of my frustration about feeling vulnerable and different, and not being able to talk about my fears to many others at the time. Perhaps in our childhood we can be forgiven for such actions, but as we grow older, or wish to make progress, we need to create better skills through communication, and the manner in which this is done will depend partly on the form of interaction.

4.6 An examination of response

Even if you consider yourself quite confident at being able to pick up the meaning of most verbal dialogue at normal speed, there may still be many occasions that could catch you unaware of how to respond suitably, and this could cause embarrassment if one is not prepared. It is not always appropriate to express your thoughts out loud. For instance, suppose you were invited to a friend's wedding, and despite enjoying it for a while you then found at the reception that they were offering you some cake that you really did not like the look or taste of. In your own mind, a comment such as 'I hate this horrible cake – take it away' may appear logical, since you are simply expressing your views on the fact that you do not wish to eat the cake. However, such comments must be resisted, as they go against what is considered acceptable and risk upsetting the provider and the other guests – after all, if you had spend a long time preparing some food for someone in advance, only for them to turn round and say 'This is terrible, get rid of it!' you would hardly be very happy. So if in a social situation you find yourself wishing to express a view about something, it pays to consider the feelings of others around you as well as your own. In the above scenario, why not say something like 'Do you mind if I leave the cake, or may I have some biscuits instead?' (if they are on offer). The more you experience different situations such as this, the more confident you will become on how to handle them in the correct manner.

It is also important not to intimidate or put unnecessary pressure on other people by making inappropriate responses or demands, even within your own family. A great many of us find considerable comfort (it may even appear essential in our own minds!) in having a rigid timetable each day, such as meals at the same time, and constant attention. However, it will not help either you or your parents if you try to rule their lives by insisting on unreasonable demands being met and threatening to run amok or to fly into a rage if they are not. Such action can both inhibit any chance of you making further progress and at the same time thoroughly wear out your parents with exhaustion. Most of us can be surprisingly adaptable (within reason) to what is allowed and permissible with, say, a set of ground rules, and will be familiar enough with our immediate surroundings to be able to follow them. It is perfectly OK to discuss a fear or anxiety with a trusted parent once, for instance. It is not acceptable to check with them a further ten times and keep waking them up in the night to do so, as I found out to my cost when I was younger! After a while of repeatedly checking the same thing with someone, you may find that the fear of that person getting annoyed with the fact that you keep asking them is greater than your fear of the original worry. An experience such as this can actually be good for you, in the sense that it can force you to think up solutions for yourself.

4.7 Being taken advantage of

There will be occasions when we can become vulnerable by taking too literally a phrase or sentence that another states, or not being aware that the person is actually trying to manipulate us to their own advantage. Often this can occur at times of the day which are less structured (such as break-time at school or college). If someone you did not know well suddenly approached you and asked you if they could borrow £2 to buy some food, there is a danger that you could agree without any reservations as, in your mind, the word 'borrow' has indicated that your money will be returned to you at some point. In reality it is far more likely that you will never see your money again and the other person has no plans on getting it back to you, just as when a bird catches a worm, it is most unlikely that it will then release the worm again. So beware of being tricked by others whom you do not feel comfortable with or do not know well enough to trust them. It is not fair on you for your teachers or parents to expect you to know at first how to deal with all the situations that can occur and if you are at all uncertain about any particular happenings you should discuss them with your parents or carers. It is a good idea to check that your parents are having regular meetings with your teachers if you feel able to ask this, because problems that develop can often be caught at an earlier stage and ironed out as they occur if your teachers are keeping an eye out for you. Moreover, regular meetings with staff members yourself can be very comforting and can offer additional ideas of aid; for example, having a communication book (a written record of rules on how to handle various situations that can be referred to when the need arises).

4.8 A method of learning social skills in a safe environment

An especially good aid to help us overcome and learn to deal with some of these social problems is within a so-called 'social skills group'; I attended one when I was younger at the Chinnor Resource Unit for autistic children, which was held once a week after normal school hours. This involved a meeting of anything up to about ten autistic people accompanied by several teachers. The aim of the meeting was to give us a chance to discuss any social difficulties that were concerning us at the time, as well as acting out role play of actual social situations that might arise in everyday life and thinking about how to deal with them. The sessions were often videoed so that they could be examined and played back later. Additionally, the mere fact that some of us were requested to perform or express our viewpoints in front of the others was an opportunity for us to relate to and get to know the rest of the group, which was good experience in itself. The group 'tasks' could also be adjusted in difficulty level according to the severity of autism in the audience, with simpler commands such as 'Go and say hello to John' to the less able; a request like 'Describe your feelings to the others on when you are bullied, and how you deal with it' would only be given to one of the more verbally fluent and confident learners among us.

4.9 What if I am not verbally fluent?

While the ability to interpret information correctly and decide on a suitable reply can be challenging even for those among us who are fluent and able in their verbal speech and understanding, let us remember those other individuals who unfortunately will not be in this position, who will perhaps have a different way of understanding. Moreover, the task of making sense of the rules of social society can be even more daunting if you are not verbally fluent, but there are forms of alternative strategies possible, which can reach and teach alternative communication systems. I once had the privilege of being able to meet a man who had effectively no verbal skills at all, and his only method of communication was through a form of touch-typing onto a keypad where the messages were then relayed onto a screen, but I thought he handled life wonderfully. For him, computer technology was not just an option, but essential for any dialogue. I managed to have quite an intelligent conversation with him about maths and the formula for solving quadratic equations. The immense smile on his face told me that he knew that I had understood his form of language and had taken the time to make a decent reply.

4.10 Alternative communication

4.10a Alternative communication 1: Computers and the Internet

The mention of computers may make some of you think of playing video games for a fun pastime, but they can also offer us the chance to learn serious work through fun and a relaxed set-up, possibly because a computer always obeys fixed rules. This could be through a challenge game, where you have to find and type in the answers to some challenging questions in order to win, or perhaps on a more basic level by having to listen to instructions from a certain software before giving a typed reply to the computer. The very fact that using a computer demands a certain amount of logic and precise understanding can appeal to many of us who generally like an ordered and structured state of affairs with our work. The Internet is an additional source where one can learn to seek out information, or even talk to others visually, although I would recommend that a trusted adult should supervise you to begin with until they are sure that you are aware of the basic dos and don'ts of being online (such as cost and avoiding inappropriate websites). It can be very useful if you have an urgent query about an assignment at school or at college to be able to use a computer to contact your tutor instantly rather than track him down physically. On the other hand it may be tempting to overdo your use of a computer so that it becomes almost an obsession. Care should be taken to avoid this by such activities as setting yourself a maximum time limit or allowance for spending on it each day, asking others to enforce it if necessary!

4.10b Alternative communication 2: The Picture Exchange Communication System

Sometimes people with autism cannot communicate directly. For instance, if a child wants a biscuit, she may take her mother to the biscuit tin. This is not a real communication. The Picture Exchange Communication System is a way of trying to help the child make a positive communication towards the person who will give her the biscuit.

Objects, pictures, words and sentences can be used to make the exchange, although in most cases the aim is to use the sentence strip and spoken language together. The sentence strip will have key words or pictures fixed to a strip of card.

For example:

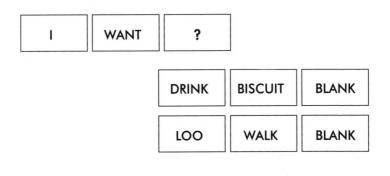

Key cards

The exchange is as follows:

- The teacher gives the strip to the learner.

- The learner has a picture collection with his favourite requests on it.

- The learner takes the picture or key word he wants and fixes it onto the sentence strip.

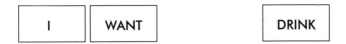

- The learner hands the entire sentence strip to the teacher.

- The teacher reinforces the exchange by repeating the message and often naming the learner, saying 'I want drink – oh James, you want a drink?'

- Teacher gives the drink to James.

Once this becomes an established pattern, it can be expanded to include all aspects of language, including correct grammatical structures. It can also include an extensive list of the learner's needs and interests. In many cases, once the learner has begun to use the exchange as a form of communication, spoken language follows more easily. This is often used with younger children, but has also been used successfully with older people with autism who have not previously found any satisfactory way of communicating.

4.10c Alternative communication 3: The Options approach

One of the most common difficulties for us when being taught is that we always seem to have to try to 'fit in' and follow rules from a bewildering and at times overwhelming world that never seems to work on our terms. However, a particularly interesting form of assistance (known as the Option Institute's Son-Rise Program) takes a different approach and involves other people attempting to enter the world as we see and think of it by copying our actions from both a verbal and a physical perspective. The basic idea of this is to make progress by seeing things from our point of view and joining with us rather than seeming to be against us. There is something comforting about this for us, and it is almost as if we have found someone familiar, in the sense that we can relate to them just like someone in a wheelchair who had just met a second wheelchair-bound person, or a deaf man meeting another deaf man, each understanding those of the other's difficulties that are similar in nature. There is evidence that when a parent or teacher imitates our own actions, it can increase the amount of interest and curiosity we experience. It feels less threatening and makes it possible for us to show more eye contact. It may also help us to be more able to learn in a less demanding situation. This activity must of course always be done in a sincere way!

The Options approach can be carried out by parents at home as well as by teachers and other staff members, but to work effectively the risk of distractions should be minimised. It is suggested that the individual be in a quiet room, perhaps with bland walls and a plain floor, with most background noise filtered out, together with gentle, even lighting. Normally, only one adult will be present for the session, and a set of toys or other objects will again be somewhere in the room out of reach, such as on a series of shelves high up on one of the walls. These items are given by the adult when they are requested. The adult present will be the person in the room who becomes the most important and interesting object for us to relate to and learn to trust. They play the central role to that effect, always seeking the chance to make a connection or communication real. This approach can have an astonishing effect on improving interaction, communication skills and confidence, even for those of us who have severe autism and anxieties, and can eliminate many of our fixations, including inappropriate movements of body and lack of eye contact.

4.10d Alternative communication 4: ABA

Another well-known intervention stemming from American research is known as ABA – Applied Behaviour Analysis. It also aims to teach us communication skills and creativity in a very structured manner, but is more intensive than the Options approach and requires most people in daily contact with the learner to be involved in order to operate successfully. ABA relies on a system of positive reinforcement. The learner is directed to complete a small task, and immediately receives a positive reward. For example, the act of sitting down. This is immediately followed by praise, which could be part of a biscuit, a thumbs-up sign or a comment like 'good boy!'. The routines are practised many times until the rewards can be gradually reduced and the positive behaviour remains. The tasks have to be very carefully matched with the level of development and understanding of the learner. In many cases, it has been found that this kind of strategy can be extremely useful for the younger learner, especially for certain basic behaviours. Once again though, this is an approach which could also help some individuals who find external reinforcement helpful, such as knowing there will be a small treat to follow a challenging task, perhaps a reward of some ice-cream following a visit to the local supermarket for the first time.

4.11 Where can I find out more?

Effective communication between us and others can be likened to an opening of the door, at least partially, to our closed world of mistrust and fear, giving us the chance to 'see the light of understanding' in the sense that we can at least express our fears to others and be comforted by any reassurance given to us. A full list of aids for autistic people is fairly extensive, and I have not been able to give anything more than a brief introduction to some of them here. A thoroughly trained team or individual teacher is often needed to try to determine which of them is most appropriate for each one of us, as it will depend on a number of factors, such as our concentration level, the predictability of our behaviour patterns and the stage of our education and social development. Further details of language therapies available can be found in local libraries or by contacting the National Autistic Society, who will also have information on appropriate computer material, although this is still in a fairly early stage of development. In addition the NAS will have information for the aids I have mentioned above and others. Please also refer to specialised books on the subject, and the Internet can also often be a good way of collecting required data. At the end of the day, remember that whichever type of assistance is used, it should be one where we feel comfortable and can be able to show at least some form of progress after a period of time. Non-verbal skills can be just as crucial in our development as verbal ones, not just when we are children, but in later life as well. The ability to write allows us to be organised, write appointments and keep diaries. It also enables us to keep records of our anxieties and how to deal with them (see Chapter 5), without speech being a constant necessity. And while fluent talking ability and understanding might be the final or ultimate goal for an autistic individual, even one or two small steps towards that goal can be considered an achievement in itself, paving the way for ever larger successes in the future.

CHAPTER 5

The Art
of Independent Living

In this chapter I shall be giving advice for those autistic individuals who have recently moved into their own accommodation (or are considering this), with only minimum support (perhaps a brief visit once a week from a rehab officer or social worker). For most people, living alone for the first time can be daunting, or at least challenging, with all the new requirements such as handling finance, home maintenance and change of location. For the autistic person this process can be even more difficult, even overwhelming at times, as countless tasks such as obtaining one's own food become the sole responsibility of the individual concerned, rather than their family or carer as previously. How then can such an individual cope without being swept away by a tidal wave of continuous anxiety?

5.1 Getting started

The first point to note, of course, is the fact that any autistic person who has come far enough in their progress of life to be even considering living alone has a right to feel pretty proud because in 'independence terms' they are about to enter the élite of the top few per cent who have sought (and in many cases achieved) becoming self-sufficient. It can be likened to a footballer having earned the right to play for his home team in the World Cup competition. If successful, that player will greatly broaden his horizons in terms of future opportunities, earn respect from others and develop a sense of intense well-being and inner confidence. However, if we want our just rewards, we will have to work for them. It is all very well when things are looking up. The real test comes when they are not. Every detail of change in moving house can matter to an autistic person, and the parts that seem the hardest often matter the most.

There is no way that anyone can ever predict every single little event that could occur through moving house that may end up challenging us or making us anxious. The trick is to recognise the ones that really matter. The fundamental rule is to have a thorough contingency plan so that you know what to do if any of these 'important' happenings occur and demand attention. Communication from others is vital for this. If the occurrence is serious or causes severe worry immediate advice from others will be necessary; this will normally be in the form of the telephone, although other forms of instant dialogue such as the Internet or going round to a friend's house to ask advice are possibilities. Less serious events causing only a moderate amount of worry can often be dealt with by having pre-written notes in a 'worry reference book', or by waiting until one sees other people. Before we discuss more on the use of these aids, we must first decide what constitutes a serious event, demanding immediate attention.

5.2 Get your priorities in order

Let us consider the fundamental requirements for people to survive in their own homes. They will need enough drink and food each week; they will need to keep warm, with lighting at night; they will need to have enough money, and be able to handle its management; and they will need to have water for washing and laundry. These requirements require electricity for heating and preparing food, providing lights and security, and mains water supply. If any of these basic requirements is cut off, action is needed quickly. Without mains power one could find oneself in a freezing cold, pitch-dark house without being able to see where anything is. Without water we cannot survive for long. Occurrences such as these would warrant a phone call within 24 hours. In extreme cases, such as a major water leak or house fire, first attempt to remove yourself from the danger, then make contact with others at once (more on this later in the chapter).

By contrast, there are many things that may catch your eye in your home, perhaps late at night, such as a set of cobwebs above your kitchen table, which would *not* warrant you phoning people up in the middle of the night, no matter how much you might be worrying about germs falling on your kitchen surface when you try to clean them up. In the daytime too, you must use some common sense. There is nothing wrong with phoning up a good friend to put your mind at rest about some minor concerns. What is not right is phoning up another 20 times on the same day every time you think of another worry! This is where having a reference book to refer to can be so vital, especially as many anxieties tend to repeat themselves. Often, as soon as we sort out one worry, another seems to come along in its place. Let us now examine the possible make-up and layout of such a book, and how it can reduce your anxieties to a number of situations.

5.3 The worry check-book

5.3a The aid of a worry check-book

There may be many things in each room of your house that could cause concern, from a loose shelf with books (will it fall?) to a front door with a defective lock, to rust forming in the kitchen sink, so it will help greatly to divide your worry check-book up into different sections, either by room or by topic. Each section should be clearly marked, perhaps with a contents listing at the front. To illustrate the method, I shall relate this to my own experience. My original use of a worry check-book stemmed from my fear of leaving electrical switches of appliances, such as the cooker, switched on by mistake, which would have resulted in a fire or things overheating. Away from the security of being able to ask my parents to check, it was now vital that I could be able to check whether a switch or knob was off or on by myself. So I proceeded with the help of a great and trusted friend to draw a picture of every main switch and knob involved with electricity in every room of my house, and what its shape looked like when both on and off.

5.3b The danger of overlooking small details

For several weeks this new system worked wonders! No longer did I have to keep ringing people up or asking them to remind me what it looked like when this and that appliance was off. Whenever I had any doubt, or could not remember, even in the middle of the night, I simply referred to my trusted notepad to put my mind at rest. I totally trusted my friend who had helped me, so I trusted the information in my notepad as well. It was not just the standard shape of a normal socket switch, but others as well. The oven knobs all had to have a pointer at number 0 to be off, and my electric shaver had to have its shiny light 'not' glowing for it to be off. By referring to these pictures, I was able to reduce my anxiety instantly, almost as if I had asked someone in person. I was gaining more confidence in this system by the day until, that is, late one evening I leant down by my cooker and happened to look at the knobs and switches from the other side. Suddenly I broke out in a cold sweat. I was shaking with fear and worry. Something had broken my sense of security!

It is almost as if autistic people can have anxieties that they are not even fully conscious of, worries that stay just below the surface, until some event triggers them off. I had always taken instruction very literally, to the extreme, and had been very particular about being accurate, especially in something like checking cooker knobs were turned off. Now I had cause for concern. I was doubting that accuracy. The problem was this: if we look at a standard switch or knob from the left-hand side, it does not look the same shape as when viewed from the right-hand side. And when my friend had been helping me draw my pictures, she had been standing on the left, and I on the right of the appliances. Filled with dismay, I realised I had drawn almost the whole set of pictures back to front. Common sense should have prevailed. Deep down I had an intuitive idea of what had happened. I had put 'from the right, switch looks like this' because I was standing on the right. And I had forgotten that my friend was telling me switch shapes from the left, because *she* was standing there! But I needed reassurance.

I phoned my friend in the middle of the night. I was that worried. She had to come round and help me redraw the pictures, more generally this time, to allow for the fact that we might look at the switches from different angles. And I then spent weeks dwelling on my apparent lack of perception and precision and how I could have failed to spot something so important in my mind earlier. Most people would not blink an eyelid over this – it would not even cross their mind. But to an autistic person such as myself such detail can be paramount. However, the point to note is that I survived! I came through the experience a stronger person, knowing not to fall into the same trap again. That is why we must never shy away from trying. We cannot expect things always to run smoothly, and there will be traps lying in wait for us. But going through these experiences and dealing with them is the only way we can reach the self-fulfilment of truly confident independence.

5.3c Improve the design of your book layout

As well as chapters on individual room worries, I also had a more general section of reference in my worry reference book. This would cover many other things which were very useful to refer to without having to phone people up. For example, how do you tell the difference between a cooking apple and an eating apple? How do you deal with a splinter or corn on your foot? And do drivers always pay for any petrol they get at garages rather than any of the passengers? Sections such as these can be added to at any time when you have asked someone a question, so that you can jot it down for future reference. Do not try to write everything at once, however. For example, when you start your check-book it is best to consider, say, the three or four things most important to you in each room first. And try to generalise a situation: for example, rather than note that this kitchen switch looks a certain way when off, consider the shape of all standard electrical switches in every room in your house. In this way we can avoid tedious repeats in every room. There will always be exceptions and two-way switches but we can make a separate note of them.

To summarise then, whenever a worry surfaces, we should categorise it into three types.

- Is the worry Type 1, a *minor* worry? This could be something like a packet of biscuits dropped on the floor or a leaky bottle of drink from the shops. What if the crumbs fell under or behind the fridge or some liquid from the drink stained the fridge – would it be safe? These are the sort of thing we could refer to our worry check-book or sort out ourselves (for example, take the drink back to the shop for a refund or replacement) without having to consult others.

- Or is it a more *major* worry, such as a total power cut or a lost purse? These are the types of things that will cause considerable inconvenience and are worth a phone call.

- Rarely, we may encounter *emergencies* such as a house fire, or a flooded house. It is a good idea to fit smoke alarms in your house, plan an escape route from the building and find out where the nearest public callbox is, or make a plan with a friend nearby to go to them in the event of a crisis. I do not approve of hiding a spare set of house keys outside your home in case you get locked out. It is the first thing a burglar will look for, so keep a spare set with a trusted friend or family member instead.

5.4 Thoughts on shopping organisation

On the topic of buying and preparing your own food: many autistic people may find it easier to go with someone the first few times, as supermarkets can often be very busy, crowded and noisy places. Until you are very confident it is a good idea to make a shopping list of your main requirements – you will have some knowledge of this from the food that you enjoyed up till now while living with your family or carers. Ticking off the items as you buy them can save a huge amount of time; other advantages of the shopping list is that you can get an idea of how much you are spending each week and whether you are having a healthy diet. You will have to decide how you will store and prepare the food at home. Do you have enough cupboards? Do you have a fridge and freezer for frozen goods? Being able to cook meals successfully can be very satisfying but it takes experience and must be done with care, since many accidents, such as getting burned, occur in the kitchen. You should always attempt cooking initially with supervision from a trusted adult or carer and should not attempt it on your own until they have given you permission.

5.5 Handling money wisely

Managing how much money you spend is an important skill to be acquired when you live by yourself. Your parents or social worker/carer will have a good idea on how much approximately you should be spending each week. As well as making shopping lists, you can keep till receipts to have accurate records. The amount you can spend will depend upon many factors, including whether you are working full or part time, or are on benefits. It is important to realise that any agreed amount to spend weekly will not be exact, for example perhaps in one week you might spend £10 extra for a friend's birthday and a day trip by train, then in the next week spend £10 less than usual by staying at home more. What matters is the overall average that you spend in the long run. You will of course sometimes like to treat yourself to a new book or video game as well as buying food, and this is often a matter of common sense – it is OK to do this now and then, but not OK to spend £80 on one-armed bandits and CDs every week.

5.6 Transport

5.6a Ways of getting about

Unless you are very lucky and live close enough to town to walk there, you will also have to consider your transport from place to place. It is not practical to rely on friends all the time, so most of us will have to either learn to drive or come to terms with public transport. While it is true that a few autistic individuals have managed to learn to drive and own a car, they are probably in the minority. For one thing it is very expensive, not just obtaining a vehicle but even having lessons. For another it is a big responsibility. Driving has to be done properly and carefully, otherwise it is dangerous, just like cooking. Any factors that could affect your concentration as a result of your disability will have to be considered. Would you panic in certain situations, such as heavy traffic or a car skid? Are your eyesight and hearing good enough? The person or people responsible for your care will give you advice on your ability to drive. If you can show that you clearly have the ability, it will give you a lot of new independence. But we have to be able to face up to the responsibility that comes with it and the consequences of our actions.

For many autistic individuals, driving themselves is not a practical or realistic option. But let us not be too negative – it is still possible to live a very fulfilling life using alternative methods of getting around. If you are very fit and able, cycling offers a cheap way of travelling locally, especially if your local area is not too hilly! Otherwise we have buses, trains and maybe sympathetic friends to give us a lift. You may even have additional private services in your area such as a 'dial-a-ride' where you can book a vehicle in advance to take you to your destination. Even if you are not near any major public services, you can always call a taxi. Let us examine in brief these different options. It is always a good idea to plan ahead and allow for extra time in case there are delays. Make sure you have a good map on you, especially if you plan on travelling outside your local area. By organising yourself before-hand for all the most likely complications of travelling, you can reduce the risk of that all-too-familiar panic attack.

5.6b Cycling (on yer bike!)

Being able to get about is a vital skill that needs to be acquired when living independently, not only for essential items such as shopping, but for a social life too. It would be a very depressing existence to sit cooped up in your home every day. Cycling, the cheapest option discussed of getting around, is of course the most vulnerable to the elements, so *do* check the weather forecast before you go out and dress appropriately. You must ensure that you are comfortable on your bike (it should be the right size), that you can ride it safely and that you are aware of the Highway Code rules for cyclists (how to signal, and understanding and obeying traffic signs). Ask an adult to advise you or take a cycling profi-ciency test. Pay particular attention to the wheels, brakes and lights on your bike and make sure they are in good working order. Remember that lights are a legal requirement for cyclists at night. As long as you are careful and have good road sense there is no reason why you cannot learn. However, if all this seems a bit too challenging, choose another option where the responsibility of driving is not yours.

5.6c Buses and trains

Buses and trains, of course, are means of transport where you are not the driver, so you can sit back and enjoy the view. But as with many things, autistic phobias can often build up. I know from my own experience that I was once petrified about the prospect of travelling on a train by myself, for fear of missing my stop and becoming stuck perhaps hundreds of miles from home. I believe that most of these so-called 'phobias' have a good reason for starting, in my case stemming from an incident when I was younger, when I could not get one of the old-style push-open train doors to open and thus had to remain on the train against my wishes. Many of these anxieties seem to lie dormant for years until almost subconsciously they are reactivated when we face a similar challenge to our security. The trick for coping is to realise that it is not all that bad. One has to get things into perspective. Most trains these days have easier push-button doors anyway. But even if it did happen, you could ask someone else to open the door at the next station and then catch the next train back. Or phone a friend for some help. Have a couple of phone numbers with you for situations like this.

5.7 Other transport considerations

You may find yourself relying on a bus or a train to get you to work or an important interview. One of the first things you will find is that both these forms of transport often do not run on time. Actually, especially in the case of buses, running exactly to the timetable is a rarity. There are just too many factors, such as heavy traffic, roadworks or bad weather, that can disrupt the schedule.

5.7a Public transport just does not connect

Not only that, but whenever one needs to make a connection from one bus to another, or perhaps from bus to train, they may seem to be magically timed to just miss one another. At the Haddenham and Thame Parkway train station on the Marylebone to Birmingham line, there is a connecting bus service to Thame and Oxford that I have used for a number of years. I say connecting, but in fact each train is timed to miss the bus by about a couple of minutes. More often than not, however, the bus tends to run about one and a half minutes late, just allowing me to see it pull away as my train pulls up at the station. The number of times this has happened to me is endless! I then have to wait for 29 minutes and 40 seconds until the next (half-hourly) bus arrives, and as I get on and it pulls away I then see the next train pulling in, with the next batch of unfortunate passengers who will then have to wait the same time again before another bus. At times I felt like screaming out of frustration. If I were a giant I could literally reach out my hand and pick up the bus, it was so close. It is no good getting a different train later or earlier. The problem occurs right through the day. The bus company just are not interested in changing their times, arguing that they have connections to make elsewhere. On Sundays it is only an hourly service, or worse. It is quicker to walk over two miles into Thame, say, than wait for the next bus after just missing one.

5.7b Another example of missed connections

I have also had plenty of fun elsewhere. That of course was an ironic comment! While reading for my BSc degree at Brunel University I required two different buses to get home – one to get me into Uxbridge, the other to get me from Uxbridge to High Wycombe. Now each lecture generally took place from five minutes past each hour until five minutes to each hour. But it was not always precisely the case. To an autistic person, even a two-minute difference can seem like an eternity. Especially when it can make over an hour and a half's difference in your time of getting home. Picture a day when my last lecture finished on time, at 4.55 p.m. I would race out of the lecture room and across the university, past the maths building, then the sports and arts centre and up to the main road and bus stop. It is hard to believe anyone could run so fast. My whole body ached, I was so exhausted I often felt like choking. I knew that a bus into Uxbridge usually came at 4.59 p.m. I had to be at the bus stop by 4.58 p.m. and 45 seconds to stand any chance. Even if I succeeded the battle was not over. The bus took about seven and a half minutes on average to reach central Uxbridge. Which left me just 30 seconds to jump off this bus, cross the road and jump on the High Wycombe bus – due to leave Uxbridge at 5.07 p.m., of course. And get me home for 6 p.m. But one slow tractor or extra set of red traffic lights and it is all over. There was the second bus driving off into the distance. It was always pot luck.

Now what about another week: same lecture, same day. But perhaps the lecturer came in a couple of minutes late and it took him an instant longer to finish. Perhaps he took a couple of minutes longer than usual handing out some leaflets. It does not really matter how it happened. The point is, it is now 4.57 p.m. There is no hope now! Sadly, I pick up my heavy bag and walk agonisingly slowly down the path. There is no point in rushing now. I shall never get the 4.59 p.m. bus into Uxbridge and consequently will never reach the 5.07 p.m. bus back to High Wycombe. That means a wait of at least an hour until 6.07 p.m. and probably more, because this bus normally gets caught in the rush hour on its way here. It could be long after 7 p.m. before I get home. Think of all the things I could have done in that time. Got my homework done so I could relax later. Had a meal and some drinks to unwind. Got some phone calls out of the way. Now, none of that is possible. I shall probably be so late that by the time I have got home and got myself settled, it will be time to go to bed. 'No favourite TV programme for me any more, despite looking forward to it all week!' I would mutter to myself. 'This spoils everything. Just everything!'

5.7c *The importance of reading timetables correctly*

What I was complaining about was my sense of helplessness with a situation beyond my control. This is a feeling that we autistic people can be very familiar with. The inadequacies of public transport can force you into a position where you have to face altering your plans or your normal schedule at short notice. This kind of unpredictability is exactly the sort of thing that can make us anxious and in a predicament. The trick is to learn how to get out of the predicament, and to be prepared for things to happen. After all, the chance of this country having a decent connecting transport system in every rural town within the foreseeable future is about as remote as seeing a green elephant from Mars! So it is up to you to conquer the transport system, before the transport system conquers you. Recently, I had a chance to put my coping strategy to the test. Having already mastered travelling to many stations on the Underground from Marylebone (a few years back), I travelled up to London on an evening when I knew that Marylebone station was closing at 10.20 p.m. (earlier than usual) because of engineering work. I had also noticed that later trains back to High Wycombe were going from Paddington station. With a little time on my hands before my meeting I thought I would go and visit it from the Underground, just in case I missed the last Marylebone train home, although I thought at the time, surely that would be very unlikely in the near future.

Later that evening I set off on the Underground on my way to Marylebone to go home. The tube arrived at Marylebone at 10.09 p.m. and 30 seconds, in good time for the 10.20 p.m. train. Or was it? What 10.20 p.m. train? I had just looked at the timetable again. I had misread the information. While it was true that the Marylebone station stayed open until 10.20 p.m., the last train to High Wycombe from there was *10.10* p.m. And here I was, still in the underground station at 10.09 p.m. and 30 seconds. This seemed a familiar situation. Just not enough time to run up the escalator. But now, instead of panicking, I was able to use my back-up plan made a few hours earlier, literally. I still vividly remembered where Paddington station was. And I was not daunted by the giant size of the station, nor the fact that I had to find my way across the other side to the right platform (in the pitch dark) for the High Wycombe train, because I had familiarised myself with the place earlier in the day. I might have been late home, but I got there in the end. I had made a decision beforehand to plan ahead and asked myself, 'What would I do if this happened?' It was a good decision and it had now reaped dividends. The art of good decision-making can be learnt only through experience. And it lies at the root of successful and confident independent living, as well as guiding us through life's challenges more easily. I would urge you too to think ahead. Plan for scenarios and situations before they happen. Do not wait until you miss the last train. *And read the small print on the timetables.*

5.7d Plan ahead

With timed appointments too, be safe. Aim for an earlier bus or train. It is better to be half an hour early than half an hour late. And make sure you are able to get back from your venue too. Be aware that by mid-evening many local services may thin out, or even stop altogether, so check the timetable carefully. When you have mastered a 'new' place and been there several times you will find more confidence and a sense of satisfaction, in contrast to the first time which can feel, in swimmers' terms, like diving straight into really cold water. However, sometimes we have to 'take the plunge' to make progress. Keep to simple destinations first, then go further afield when you feel up to it.

The London Underground, for those not familiar with it, can be quite a daunting place, even for non-autistic people, but once again a seemingly impossible goal can become possible to achieve if done properly. Why not try to find your way round initially (with a good map) with a friend with you who will help if you get stuck? Then try going to exactly the same destinations on your own. Finally, explore the network at your leisure! Remember there will always be inspectors and other people in authority who will help you if you do get lost. You may also find that having a wish to go somewhere can override your fear of the unknown. Maybe a show or event in London that you have really wanted to go to for ages or, as in my case, a longing to see a great friend I had not seen for years. My wish to be reunited with this friend was greater than my fear of travelling to an unknown Tube station to find her. Most major places in the country are within reach of some Tube, train or bus, and this will greatly increase your chance to get out and about, meet more people and have fun!

5.8 Other forms of transport

As for the other options, your local library should have information on any extra services (such as dial-a-ride) that may run in your area. Read their rules of conduct carefully, the times they operate, and where they pick up/set down people. Catching a taxi is another option. However, you need to be aware that this normally costs a great deal more than the other forms of transport. You should make sure that you have enough money on you at all times when travelling, but with taxis this is especially important. Taxi rates are often increased late in the evening, or at weekends and public holidays, and even a two-mile trip can cost over £10. Many taxi drivers expect a tip (extra money for the trip), others do not like it if you do not give the right change. Many people have different views on how much to tip. It might be an extra 10 per cent, a bit more, a bit less, or even no tip at all. It is exactly this sort of grey area of uncertainty that autistic people can find stressful. It is safer usually to catch a 'registered' cab (with a number on top of the vehicle) or find a reliable firm that has the approval of a trusted friend.

The world of public transport does not seem to be particularly helpful to autistic people's reassurance! Bus and train drivers are not always sympathetic. But it is likely that you will have to face these challenges at some point in your life. Sometimes, of course, you may be lucky enough to get a lift to a place from your friends or carers. This can be very helpful at times, but it should not be relied on always. Remember that the ultimate goal of independence is to stand on your own two feet. If we get too used to people giving us lifts, we may struggle more when they are not around. I shall be covering more on accepting lifts from friends and getting to venues in the next chapter. But now, having considered getting about outside and some general rules on checking your home is safe, let us consider the task of actually maintaining your home in good order and keeping it clean. Exactly how much housework does one have to do? We do not wish to live in dirty homes, with papers and shoes all over the floor ready to be tripped over, and dirt all over the eating area. But neither do we want to be stuck at home all day every day cleaning things. So how can we get the balance right between caring too much, and not caring enough?

5.9 I hate housework! How do I deal with it productively?

Generally speaking it is better to do small amounts of housework, more often, instead of trying to do everything at once. For example, why not clean the kitchen sink and bathroom once or twice a week instead of leaving it for a month and finding it covered in deep-set rust that takes ages to clear? By cleaning more regularly you can prevent substantial dirt from building up, and thus the task can be done quicker. Often it is a case of using your common sense. If you suddenly notice your work table looking very dusty then clean it, but there is no point in cleaning something just for the sake of it if it already looks clean. Remember that you must take responsibility for most of the jobs of keeping the house clean, such as hoovering, sweeping and washing up. Try to avoid leaving objects such as shoes in doorways and other places where you might trip over them – many household accidents have occurred in this way. Do make sure you have enough goods at home for your needs. Do not wait until Sunday for example, then decide to do some cleaning, only to find you are out of cleaning products and you cannot get to the shops to buy more.

A particularly good time to clean the house is the day before you have guests or friends round, especially the hall and lounge, and rooms they may be spending time in. After all, imagine if the roles were reversed – would you prefer to visit a nice clean inviting house, or a dirty run-down one with shoes and bags all over the floor? You will also have to decide how to do your washing – you might go to the launderette or have a washing-machine at home. I must confess I'm happier with the launderette. As with almost everything else, if I fear a washing-machine flooding, I could feel compelled to sit in the house watching the machine run its full cycle, unable to do anything else! It even got to the extent when I would carry my heavy washing-bag two miles each week for a service wash rather than face the fear of flooding. Autistic people can go to extraordinary lengths to avoid stressful situations. Sometimes we can avoid them, or make alternative plans which are easier. But there are times when we have to face them, to make further progress in our lives. Being able to distinguish these different cases is an important part of becoming a more confident person living independently.

5.10 Interpreting instructions in the right way

One of the chief difficulties that autistic people have is in taking things too literally, both in the physical and written sense. I once got very concerned after leaving some toilet cleaner in the loo for 18 minutes and then flushing before realising the instructions stated not to flush for at least 20 minutes. Then my worry mode had got into gear. What if now the cleaning substance would make the loo worse? What if I damaged it or the surrounding pipes in some way, so that the toilet would break? While it is of course good practice to read the instructions on the product, I needed to realise in this case that these requirements were not that precise, and the difference between 18 minutes and 20 minutes was not significant enough to be concerned. At the time though, before one knows better, to a time-conscious autistic person this difference can seem almost infinite! Another example of how experiencing these things can teach us when to take instructions exactly and when to relax a little. One further point – it is a good idea to have some first-aid products in your house, such as plasters, in case little accidents do occur. Remember, however, these are precautionary measures: we do not have to live every moment in fear of what might never happen, just be prepared if it does.

5.11 Necessity is the mother of invention

I have spent some time explaining some of the difficulties that can occur with living independently, but we should always remember that the human being can be surprisingly effective at survival when the need arises. The saying 'necessity is the mother of invention' is perhaps appropriate here, because running your own home will force you to face situations that need resolving on your own. This is not to say of course that you can do everything by yourself. There will be larger household jobs, perhaps repairs to a damaged roof or wall or leaking pipe, where you will need help from others. But often the sheer feeling of contentment of resolving a situation yourself is worth the challenge it presents. In a strange way, knowing other people are there might make a situation more complicated. On a number of evenings I have been more relaxed at 11 p.m. than 9 p.m., since at the earlier time I would have the option of phoning others when a problem arose, whereas at the later time a feeling of inner strength would occur, so that I would not have to bother people with trivial worries, but would cope on my own since it would be too late to phone them anyway.

Even today, there are still things that can catch me out living in my own home, but I have learnt to live with them. I used to dwell on things repeatedly. I used to have a helper to mow my lawn, but would worry about the cables being trodden on, or would go to the outside store cupboard six times afterwards to make sure the mower was definitely unplugged. This sort of trap is easy to fall into, but it can consume a huge amount of unnecessary energy. Did I lock that door? Have I shut the bathroom window? The practical solution initially is to write it down on a piece of paper or make a record of the fact that the item has been checked, with the date on. Once you get more confident, you will be able to trust your instincts and memory after just checking once. We can never expect everything to always go smoothly, because life is not like that. But we can prepare ourselves as best as we can for the unexpected, and meet challenges as they arise.

CHAPTER 6

Rules of Socialising

In many ways, being able to socialise confidently is the ultimate challenge for the autistic person, who by the very definition of the condition finds the prospect of learning a mind-boggling array of different rules that seem to be different for every person. Worse still, for individuals like us, who tend to take things literally, people in society do not always mean what they say or do as they say. The more 'able' autistic individual who has the ability to carry out some communication with others but appears vulnerable is perhaps more likely to encounter bullying, or be taken advantage of, than the more severely disabled person, who is perhaps receiving help from adults all the time and thus will not come into contact with situations like these in the first place. Even the typical youngster in society would not expect to know all social etiquette at once. They would have to learn gradually through experience, just like a tennis player who starts as a novice and works his way up to a champion serving those aces. In order to make progress, we have to have those experiences, and that means taking some chances. Although we cannot predict exactly how events might turn out, there are a number of basic rules that we can follow to make us feel safer. Let us examine these.

6.1 Feeling comfortable with the situation

Clearly, it is often easier to start attending social events with someone you know very well, such as a family member or relative, who will be able to provide support with any anxieties that surface. You will be able to pick up tips on interacting with others by observing how your companion is acting and talking to others. It is also likely that you would get a lift to and from the venue in this case. Otherwise you might go with a good friend of the family after your mum or dad has agreed. You will need to feel at least fairly comfortable about the situation – always trust your instincts and if in doubt avoid the situation, at least until you have sought extra advice. For example, do not be tempted by a stranger to go with them because of promises of 'special treats' or because they say they know your mum and dad. You should wait until you can actually ask one of your parents (or your carer) if it is OK. If the person asking you is genuine, they will understand why you are checking things in this way.

6.2 Meet in public places to start with

The basic rule to follow when first getting to know someone or meeting them properly for the first time is probably to arrange a meeting in a public place, such as a shopping precinct, restaurant in town or day centre. In this way, you are much less likely to find yourself in a vulnerable situation where someone can take advantage of you, since there are likely to be a lot of other people around. And do not give out your address and phone number, even if they ask for it, unless you are totally sure you can trust them. If things do not work out, it is then easier to back out of the situation, whereas if things do work out, you could get to know them better with a few more meetings first and then give your details out. Think carefully about what time of day to make the meeting as well, and make sure the place is open at that time. There is no point in getting together with someone for a sandwich only to find the place closing in five minutes' time, leaving you both stuck outside in the pouring rain and hungry. It is also more likely you will be closer to public transport or a phone if you choose to meet in public meeting-places, should the need for help arise.

6.3 Dress appropriately for the occasion

In my own experience, until very recently, I had almost no dress sense at all. I used to put the same old holey jogger bottoms on, no matter where I went, from a casual meeting with a friend to a business meeting or interview or to a posh restaurant! Until I was told otherwise, I did not know any better. It was only when I started going out more and experiencing different events that I realised how important dressing appropriately is to creating a good impression, not just for myself but for my friends and others around me. These days I could hardly give an international level talk on autism and feel comfortable without wearing a proper outfit and nice suit. For many social meetings, dressing 'smart casual' is a good guide: a proper pair of trousers and nice top or shirt, but you might want to add a jacket in cold weather or a tie for an interview. Make sure you can put them on properly as well (or get a friend to show you). There is no point in having the right clothes and then having your collar inside out, or your tie on back to front. Because every case is different, if you are at all unsure, check with a friend or the person inviting you. Remember that at family events and social get-togethers dress sense can be particularly important.

6.4 Do not take things too literally

One of the most important things to learn about meetings and the things that friends might tell you, is not always to take them too literally. Take, for example, the supposed time of your get-together. Suppose you had arranged to meet someone you know at 4 p.m. outside the local café in your town. To many autistic people with a fixation on time, 4 p.m. means 4 p.m. exactly, that is to say 4 p.m. and no minutes and no seconds. In everyday life, however, 4 p.m. means approximately 4 p.m., even though it is not specifically stated. Thus we do not push the panic button if it is now 4.01 and there is still no sign of the friend. In fact, I would not be at all concerned if they showed up any time between 3.50 and 4.10. Remember that they, like you, will have to make their way to the meeting-place, perhaps by public transport, which may be delayed. Maybe their watch is a bit slow, or yours is a bit fast. Or perhaps they got held up in a previous meeting and could not contact you to let you know because they were not aware of it until the last minute. Equally, you would expect them to understand if you got held up by a few minutes. So be prepared for things not always going exactly as planned.

6.5 Be prepared for the unexpected

Consider again the situation of meeting the friend above, but now suppose it is 4.20 and there is still no sign of them. Now you probably have the right to feel curious about what has happened. What can you do? It will not help you to get in a panic or remain in the same place for the rest of the day. This is not practical. Think carefully about the situation. Have you definitely got the right day? And have you got the right meeting-place, or perhaps there is another café just up the road a bit further that your friend thought you meant. Even if it is definitely this café, many buildings can have more than one entrance and one exit. Maybe your friend is waiting for you on the other side of the shop.

This is why it is important to be clear about details like these beforehand, especially if you are not totally familiar with the area: for example, do not just say 'at the café', but 'by the front entrance to the café'. If you know your friend's number or mobile (you should have it on you if you do) the most obvious thing to do is to find a phone box and call them about 4.30 to find out what has happened. Have some money on you for the phone call as well (or a phone card). If things get difficult (if you cannot get through or you do not know them well enough to have their number) you may have to 'abandon ship', so to speak, and go home. Waiting half an hour for them arriving from locally should be enough. If they are coming from further afield, you might give them a little longer, say up to an hour. You could phone one of your other friends when you get home to ask their views on the matter. But at the end of the day you did your bit by showing up for the meeting. Do not assume they did not show up on purpose. Maybe they just forgot, mistook the date or had a pressing family emergency to attend to. If the person involved knows you well enough, or the meeting was important enough, they are bound to get in contact with you anyway. Otherwise it is probably not worth worrying over.

6.6 Respecting people's boundaries

Whenever we form new friendships we have the chance to have a great deal of fun and enjoyment, going to the cinema, theatre or social club, to name a few enjoyable things to do. However, it is very important to realise that your friends have their own lives to live too. You might, for example, see a friend every second Saturday, but not more than that, since they are working. Or you might phone another friend once a week for a natter on a Wednesday, since this is their day off and they are usually in a good frame of mind. Exactly how often you see someone will depend on a number of factors, such as how close they live to you, how close a friend they are, how busy they are (do they work full time, etc.), and what other commitments you have. The fact that these things can vary from person to person can make this difficult for us, but a friend will usually provide clues such as 'I'm available after next week', or 'I'm quite busy for the next fortnight'. The latter of these two statements is a polite way of saying that seeing you again will be difficult during this period. You must respect this. After all, put yourself in the reverse position – would you want to carry on seeing a friend if you were tired, did not feel well, or had stacks of assignments or work to do with a tight deadline?

6.7 Who contacts whom?

There are many subtle traps to fall into unless one is prepared, even in the simple act of telephoning a friend and asking them if they wanted to meet. I once made a mistake over this: once, about lunchtime, I managed to catch my friend in, but she was rather busy at that precise moment, so she promised to call me back later in the afternoon. I then proceeded to wait in the whole afternoon and most of the evening, cancelling a planned shopping trip and walk, for fear of appearing rude if I was not at home to answer the call. The call never came, at least not on that day, as my friend had had a pressing emergency at work, had to go out and had forgotten her promise. I soon realised that if someone says they will call you back and does not, the world goes on! We cannot stop everything we planned to do just in case of a call we might get, especially if it is only a matter of friends discussing the latest gossip. These days many phones enable you to leave messages (it is a good idea to have one yourself, then even if you are out important callers can leave you recorded news). If you know and trust the person, there is no reason why you should not make the first call or leave a message. You might then try them once more two or three days later if you have not heard back. But use your common sense! Trying ten times is unnecessary. Ultimately it is up to them to get back to you and make you an offer on meeting up if they are interested.

6.8 Meeting people with common interests

It can be immensely helpful on occasions to meet people who have similar interests to your own. You might join a club, such as an astronomy society that has regular meetings, or if you like sport you may meet people through playing games. Often you can forget all about your shyness as you discuss the latest happenings of your favourite activity. Courses and clubs exist to serve almost any interests, from needlework to clay modelling, to karate or tennis. Information about such places can be found in your local library, on the Internet or in telephone books such as the Yellow Pages. It is worth remembering as well that many clubs have extra activities once you have joined, such as social evenings and events that will give you even more opportunities to meet others and expand and improve your social skills and confidence. Remember, though, to check how much membership would cost (you may be able to get discounted rates if you are on low income) and whether you are able to get to your chosen place when required if you cannot drive yourself.

6.9 Attempt progress at a sensible pace

The complex challenges of socialising are too much to allow you to grasp them totally all at once. I would suggest that in the beginning, when you are only just starting to improve your confidence by meeting others, you ought to keep things simple and fairly short. Why not simply meet up for a coffee for half an hour, or perhaps go to something like a church service one morning if you get the chance? Such places often run a number of activities for people to get together and involved in as well as singing and prayers. You may know a member of your family who attends church or other social functions regularly, who could invite you to come along with them. The other advantage of going with someone you really know or meeting friends in the daytime is that you will always be able to ask advice from others, either directly or by telephone, if things do make you anxious. It is not as easy to do this if, after a night out, you are worried coming home at two in the morning, after clubbing in London, say. So it is best to wait until you really trust your friends and feel comfortable with them before staying out really late without any support. When that trust is there, however, an evening out can be a very rewarding experience.

It is important to realise that there is an enormous range of possibilities which will enable you to have a great time with your friends. For daytime activities, you might consider a visit to the sports centre to keep fit, clothes shopping in the local town, watching your favourite film at the cinema or a social event at your local village hall. Evening outings (when you are a little bit more confident) might include dining out in restaurants (more on this shortly), a night watching a show at the theatre or clubbing at the nearest facility provided for those that like to dance the night away! The next step up from a night out could be a day trip, when you might go out with your friend for a whole day. This could be to visit a theme park such as Alton Towers or a trip to the Science or Natural History museums in London. Remember, though, that outings like these require careful planning, from knowing how to get there and back again (by public transport if necessary), to how much it will cost, to organising your time. Can you be confident that your friend will be able to reassure you, not just when things are going well, but if you drop a drink all over your new trousers and get upset by this for a moment? Otherwise, you are stuck with them anyway for the rest of the day! If in doubt, aim for an easier, more 'local' encounter first.

6.10 Holidays can throw up extra tests of your coping ability

Going on holiday with someone can be even more challenging unless you really know and trust them totally. Remember that you will have to get used to unfamiliar surroundings and routine, as well as having to 'fit in' and compromise. For example, you may know the type of games or leisure activities your friend likes when you have seen them briefly in the daytime, but they might generally go to bed two hours later than you and could keep you awake with the TV on loudly for half the night. You must feel able to communicate effectively with the other person and to be able to negotiate, when necessary, when and what to do with your time.

This will stop phobias building up in your mind, as help from, say, your parents could be far away. Do not get me wrong, I do not want to be a killjoy. A week's holiday by the sea can be a wonderful experience when spending it with a caring understanding friend, but we should be under no illusion: trust of the other person and their ability to cope with you in 'worry mode' must be there to avoid upsets.

6.11 Sometimes fate determines which friendships we develop

A small number of autistic adults appear to have overcome a great many obstacles to socialising confidently, managed to meet a really good friend, perhaps starting living together, or even have a romantic relationship or get married. I shall not be examining the latter two events mentioned since I have never experienced them. But countless other people are still very lonely and are wishing for any sort of friend. The trouble is, the harder you look for them, the less chance you seem to have of finding them. Then when you least expect it, perhaps at some social function or event, you see someone who appears kind and sympathetic. Although there may be a few autistic individuals who do not wish others to know about their disability, I am in favour of telling them because more often than not, they will be very understanding and interested to know more. So just 'be yourself' and relax. There is no need to try to put on a front, so to speak, that you are really like someone else. In addition, if we try to keep ourselves busy, then we shall not have too much time to worry about being lonely when our friends are not around.

As a youngster I hardly socialised at all, even with meetings involving my own family (including cousins) and their best friends. On one occasion, a tried and trusted friend who had known my parents and me for many years came up to me asking, 'Hello Marc! How are you? I haven't seen you for a while'. I had no interest whatsoever at the time in engaging in a long conversation and, not remembering her name, simply replied, 'Who are you?' The poor lady was visibly upset, looked tearful and blurted out 'How dare you! How dare you say that to me! How could you possibly have forgotten who I am?' At the time, I simply wondered what all the fuss was about, and was unable to comprehend that not remembering a person's name (because I hardly talked to them) could offend people. My advice to others would be to learn through this experience and not make the same mistake that I did. If you see family members quite often, try to familiarise yourself with their names or write them down and make a note of them for future reference. This is especially important for those relatives (or friends in general) who may be just getting to know you or who do not fully understand your condition. It is usually OK to ask a friend's name twice, but make a note on paper after this to avoid repeatedly asking them, which may appear strange.

6.12 Respect the person's age

Age is another very sensitive area where the autistic individual can be caught unaware and act inappropriately if not forewarned. For many people, their age is a very personal thing and not something that they expect you to ask them. This particularly applies to ladies between about 40 and 60. Perhaps ladies in this age range wish to be young again, or to appear to be, and maybe those over 60 have passed the stage of being conscious about it, but whatever the reason, if in doubt *do not* ask, or check with your support worker of family member (such as a parent) for advice first. Mind you, telling a lady she is looking good is very likely to please, but not too many compliments, just one or two. However, even here, one has to be careful. One would not for example say to your friend, 'I love your grey hair!' Most people see grey hair as a sign of getting older, something they wish to avoid, so they do not need reminding of it!

6.13 Diet

6.13a Consider the implications of a diet and fitting in with others

There is one important factor that I have not yet mentioned which can have implications on our ability to fit into the social world and that is our diet, especially if this is a restricted one. It is fairly common for autistic people to latch onto a very restricted range of foods and then become very accustomed to these, to such an extent that they have no wish to try anything else. I myself was, until very recently, guilty of this, and from an early age my only cooked meal of the day consisted of two sausages and a portion of chips. I did have a few cold items as well, such as peanuts, cereals and the occasional apple, but never any eggs, milk, vegetables and the sort of things that a young child would be expected to eat. Despite this, my body appeared to have a strange metabolism and was somehow obtaining most of the nutrients I required. In these earlier years I had little or no concept of the fact that it was 'unusual' to stick to sausages and chips on Christmas and Easter Day, because I hardly ever mixed with other people. I knew of someone like me who lived on virtually nothing but baked beans every day. I could see no reason to change, just as when we are walking in the street and it is not raining, we do not see any need to put up an umbrella.

6.13b The need for adjustment

About three years ago I suddenly started having opportunities to go out socialising with people, and the restricted diet became very noticeable to my friends. After all, it is hardly normal to go to a posh restaurant for an evening meal, and then have no starters or dessert, only a main course consisting of sausages and chips. Actually it is virtually impossible! I was travelling to places such as museums in London, cinemas and amusement arcades but I was still depending on my tried and trusted formula for food. Sometimes my friends had to look for hours for a food shop or café that sold what I needed, and this often spoiled the evening. For the first time in my life I was suddenly feeling like the odd one out with everyone else tucking into roast chicken, or egg and bacon, or fish, or a hundred other items I had never heard about. But it is tough trying to change a habit you have had for years, even decades. In my mind a battle of wills was going on. Do I try new things to fit in or do I stay the same? A few months later I had decided.

It was through my tennis club in High Wycombe that I first met a really kind lady called Rosemary who had invited me out to dinner. Just a few years beforehand I never thought I would be able to socialise properly at all, and being confident enough to go dining with someone felt like a dream. For the first time I can remember my wish to 'fit in' with others was stronger than my apprehension about risking trying something new to eat. We had decided to go to 'Ask', a local restaurant in High Wycombe, for my first attempt, which was to try some salad (lettuce, cucumber, tomatoes, etc.). I knew I had tried a tiny bit of the green stuff when I was a small boy with my dad, so I knew if I had managed it then I could now. I took my first mouthful of greens. It tasted a bit strange initially, but after a few more mouthfuls I soon got used to the taste. It was certainly edible! And while I was in the restaurant I did not feel autistic or timid at all. It was almost as if I had been transformed to a more confident person and had been doing this all my life.

6.13c Branching out on new food items

From this one humble beginning many more outings with Rosemary followed, with me making more and more progress diet-wise as I was trying foods I had never dreamt I would ever have. Many of them were items I never knew existed just a few months earlier. I widened my range of salads to include the likes of radishes, onions and spring onions, peppers and mushrooms. Then I tried some pizza and pineapple, before taking a substantial liking to Chinese food, including not just items like rice, noodles, fish and prawn crackers, but also more daring choices, such as squid and octopus, as well as scallops, prawns and pakchoi. After a while I was trying things that some of my other friends were not brave enough to try! We also extended our locations of outings and meals. On one occasion we even went up to the prestigious Embassy night club in Mayfair, London, where I tried some mozzarella cheese and tomato, before dancing the night away – another first for me. All these outings were giving me a great deal of confidence and I was able to use these experiences with new foods and the knowledge that I was able to eat them to help me 'fit in' with my other friends as well as Rosemary.

6.13d The lessons to be learnt

The moral of my story here is that it is possible to break the habit of a restricted diet and become much more flexible and have a far greater choice of places to go to eat and socialise. You cannot expect to be transformed immediately, and the body may take time to adjust. One thing you may find (I certainly did) is that you can feel full up very quickly when trying new items, especially things like pizzas. So be sensible: why not just order a small portion first time? It is better to order too little (you can always order more) than too much and waste half of it. Remember also that many foods have to be eaten several times before you get used to the taste, so do not be surprised if you are undecided or something tastes strange to begin with. When I first started eating salads I found I could consume them, but after a while I began getting used to the flavour and actually started enjoying them. Inevitably there will of course be some foods that you definitely will not like. Others you will be able to eat but you will find they have a rather neutral or bland taste. The point is, even if you end up liking only a quarter of the types of food you try, you then have that knowledge for life that you can eat those things again when available in social situations.

6.13e It helps to talk through any details of an outing about which you are unsure

There are some additional complications that I still have trouble with; for example, I have not quite managed how to use chopsticks properly! There are many fine details that are not often explicitly stated but are supposed to be the norm when eating in restaurants, such as whether to eat items with a spoon, or knife and fork, and even the issue of who pays the bill at the end of the evening is a subtle one which depends on circumstances. If you are going out with the same friend frequently, you may decide to take it in turns: you pay for the meal one week and then your friend pays the next time you meet. Or you may decide to split the cost each time: perhaps you might pay for the drinks and starter, and your friend for the main course and pudding, or vice versa, and so on. If you are at all unsure about who is paying, then discuss it with your friend. Do not forget to check the prices on the menu before you order! Do not wait until after you have eaten it and suddenly find you have ordered food worth £20 more than you have between you!

It is important to stress the importance of honesty in the sort of social situations that I have been referring to here. There is no point in struggling to eat every last bit of food on your plate if you are feeling unwell or are clearly totally full up. On the other hand if a new item of food just tastes a bit strange or does not seem absolutely delicious, it is often worth persevering with it – you may get to like it. So try to use your common sense. Ask yourself, am I really feeling uncomfortable? We all have to make compromises in social occasions when our favourite items are not available. And whenever we feel able to, we should have the ability to experiment. Even if we are not feeling up to it, be tactful. A remark such as 'I hate this food, it's all gooey and trash' might be hurtful to someone who has gone to considerable trouble to set up the meeting and meal. A comment such as 'I think you've been very kind to order all this for me, I appreciate that. I am finding it very filling, do you mind if I leave a bit?' might be more productive. In addition you should find you will collect bits of knowledge in your own mind each time you experience eating out, such as the fact that drinking three lemonades before you eat can fill you up before your meal. Or the fact that Chinese restaurants tend to serve their food in small portions – useful, as you can pick and choose several items without getting full up on just one or two. As your confidence increases you will feel more and more able to rise to the challenge and excitement of trying new foods.

CHAPTER 7

Further Education and Training Survival Guide

In the eyes of many, school work can seem demanding enough, so for many people with autism, the thought of embarking on higher-level work, perhaps at a college or polytechnic – or even going to university and graduating with a degree – may seem like a distant dream which is always beyond reach. But provided you can demonstrate you have the necessary talent and potential, it is no more challenging than doing something like learning to live independently in your first flat, after relying on your family to look after your well-being until then. Sometimes we have to really push ourselves to take the 'initial plunge', so to speak, in making a big decision to go for something or aim for a big goal in life. This can take guts, especially if we do not know the outcome of our efforts. But it is always better to try. Do not fall into the trap of thinking that 'because I'm autistic I wouldn't be able to manage a higher course'. And do not let other people tell you have no chance either. There is never any harm in making enquiries about whether a particular establishment may consider a place for you. The worst that can happen is that they do not; you will have the satisfaction of knowing you tried your best and that it was not meant to be. And if there is even a one per cent chance that they will accept you, then that is still better than having no chance at all (if you do not try) of obtaining a great academic achievement and improving your self-esteem and opportunities in life for ever more. Let me also make it clear to the reader that while I have related much of the information in this chapter to my own experiences as a graduate, it can be applied to any form or standard of courses for those aged over 16 that an autistic individual may undertake, be it a science- or sports-related course, or a more unusual form of study such as hairdressing!

7.1 How do I get started?

Having made the decision to enquire and consider possible courses at post-school level, how do you then go about it? You must first be honest with yourself. What subjects would you wish to study? Are you qualified enough? Can you be sure you would be able to stick with it for several years even when the going gets tough and through examination periods? What are the practicalities of your chosen location in terms of travelling and financial considerations? And what would you wish to do after the course? Many students these days take out loans (borrow money to pay for their course expenses and then pay the money back afterwards by finding a job). The situation on these factors will depend upon individual circumstances, your own disability and how it can affect you, and the nature of the course being followed. You will also have to decide if you wish to 'live in', that is live on or near the campus throughout the duration of your course, or to remain at home and commute. I shall shortly be examining these factors in more detail, but first let me say that we need to show other people that we are serious about really wanting to give it a go. We can do this by taking the time and trouble to contact the establishments concerned, examine prospectuses, discuss financial aids and fill out forms if necessary, and attend interviews.

7.2 Consider carefully the type of course that appeals to you

The obvious initial thought is exactly what type and level of course you would like to be on. Your course may lead to the award of a diploma, A-level or perhaps an access course to allow entry for a future degree. Most prospectuses will have a number of different courses all running under one subject. You need to study the description of each course very carefully for details of work content, methods of examination and entry requirements. Mathematics, for example, may conjure up visions of algebra and trigonometry, but there are loads of different courses available, including maths with statistics, maths with finance, maths with computing and maths with language skills such as French. So consider which elements appeal most to you. Some subjects at college or university have a 'common core' of overlapping topics in each course in the first year, so if you are undecided on your main areas of interest at the start of your studies, it may be possible to transfer to another course after Year 1 when you have a better idea of the parts you wish to concentrate your studies on. Your individually obtained prospectus will have the details of this and how to apply for courses. Whatever you decide, your chosen subject clearly should be one that you have a genuine interest in and wish to know more about.

7.3 Ask yourself 'Am I qualified enough?'

You have to consider next whether you have the required academic qualifications to be eligible for the course concerned. If the level of your planned study is relatively basic, such as for further A-levels or a diploma, you may find you already have most if not all of the qualifications that you need. At the other end of the ability range, some people think that you can go to university only if you have a certain minimum number of A- or AS-levels, but this is often not the case as there are several alternative ways of gaining entrance. Such alternatives could be through an access course taken elsewhere, as a mature student or by undergoing a foundation year (an extra year) at your chosen university to help bring your work standard up to that required at degree level. You may be asked to sit a short entrance assessment or produce a short piece of work to demonstrate your suitability for the course. It is very likely that you will be asked for an interview anyway before being accepted for any course. This is your chance to 'sell yourself' and describe your abilities, but also a chance to listen to the staff on exactly what the study involves. Do arrive in good time for such a meeting and do dress respectfully – it will create a much better impression and may boost your chances of being accepted.

7.4 Think about your financial situation. Do you have enough money?

Just as with entrance requirements, so too financial situations must be considered. For many people, the idea of taking out a loan or going into debt could put them off applying in the first place, but there are many instances where autistic individuals can receive extra financial support for their study expenses, rather than relying on their families or themselves. Provided that students can show that their autism means paying extra money to attend their course, they can apply for a disabled student's allowance from their local education authority. This can give financial support for a number of things, such as travel expenses and major equipment such as computers. You may have to seek out medical proof of your disability to satisfy the local education authority that you do qualify for your allowance (your doctor could write a letter on your behalf to that effect) as well as undertake a needs assessment to establish exactly how your studies might be affected by your disability, so you have to be prepared for some form filling! If you succeed, remember it is a good idea to insure valuable items of equipment in case they are lost or stolen, and you can use some of your allowance to help pay the extra cost involved in doing this.

Even if you are unsuccessful in your claim for financial support the first time around, you may be able to get other forms of assistance. These could include access and hardship funds, opportunity bursaries or a grant. In exceptional circumstances you may be entitled to social security benefits. The rules on whether or not you can claim these different types of aid are quite complicated and depend on the individual concerned and their personal situation; full discussion cannot be given here. However, detailed information can be readily obtained from the relevant source. Good starting contacts include Skill (National Bureau for Students with Disabilities), the DRC (Disability Rights Commission) and the NFAC (National Federation of Access Centres). Once you have an idea of how much money you have coming in, you will then need to sit down and work out carefully how much you are expecting to spend per month on items not covered by allowances, a social life and basic living costs. Try to keep an accurate and clearly accessible record of your finances and update it regularly. Managing your money in a responsible way is an important skill to learn while attending a higher educational course.

7.5 Make staff aware of your condition

When you first start attending a higher education course, it will be highly desirable that *all* staff members involved with you are made aware of your condition. You may be assigned a personal tutor who will assist you when necessary throughout the duration of your course on both academic matters and those of a personal nature. Most establishments also have a disability adviser, and I would strongly recommend that you inform this person about your disability on commencing your course. They will be able to offer extra assistance for you, not only in helping you in your claim for DSA (Disabled Student Allowance) and other financial aids, but also in making contact and working together with social workers and academic departments to make life easier during your studies. They can also help by making recommendations for special considerations and take a sympathetic approach at times you find difficult, such as exams or complex coursework assignments. This could involve things like allowing extra reading time, help and supervision with precise manual work, or a special format of exam paper, such as Braille or large print.

Many autistic people I have known have been concerned that they may be treated less favourably by their place of study if they do reveal their condition, but rest assured that you can inform the disability adviser in complete confidence. Moreover, establishments are obliged to make any adjustments (within reason) to ensure that people with autism are not at a significant disadvantage compared to other students, and they are breaking the law if they fail to do so. I also found it very useful to have my personal tutor informed about my autism. I was treated very supportively and would have regular meetings with my tutor about once a week to discuss and deal with any phobias or worries that concerned me. This frequent way of dealing with anxieties proved crucial to my overall success in the course. Most students may expect to meet their tutor only once or twice a term. I attended a full-time three-year BSc, but you may decide that studying part-time or at a more basic level of work may be easier to handle, perhaps if you have a lot of other commitments, tire easily or are commuting a long way to attend lessons. You should note that a part-time course would need completing in at most twice the length expected of the same full-time course, in terms of being eligible to claiming DSA.

7.6 Consider the factors of travelling and accommodation while on your course

On the subject of travel, you have to weigh up carefully how much this could affect your studies and whether it is better to live near or on campus or to commute from where you live now. For many autistic people the stress of moving house and changing over to unfamiliar surroundings is challenging enough on its own, but this in combination with the other demands of study life, such as sorting out and learning to live with what accommodation is available on site, may be too great and they will prefer to remain in their current home or with their family. This does have the advantage of having a place to come back to that you are totally familiar with and feel safe in, but it has disadvantages as well, especially if you cannot drive. It will probably limit the number of possible options on different establishments to attend, may restrict social life in the evenings and could be very tiring. You also have to consider transport costs if these are not covered by an allowance. If you cannot face the thought of any alternative at the time, however, this may be your best option. I myself decided to commute from High Wycombe. Only two places offering the course I wanted were within feasible distance of public transport, and of the two I chose Brunel in Uxbridge. If you decide to commute you must plan your travel details carefully and learn to live with them and the restrictions they impose.

On the other hand, living on campus has the great advantage of no travelling and being within easy reach of the college or university facilities, but it may not always be possible. Although places of research generally put disabled people's accommodation on a high priority, the fact that an individual can be affected by travelling long distances and require medical aid is not necessarily a guarantee of a place available on site. Any offers made will depend on several factors, such as the severity and nature of your disability in terms of how much it would affect your performance were you not to be accommodated, and also whether anything suitable is actually available. Even if you are made an offer you will have to consider carefully exactly how independently you can support yourself. You may, for example, require the help of a care manager or personal assistant in your day-to-day chores such as dressing and feeding. If this is the case, you should discuss your requirements with your current carer or local social services department, as they hold responsibility for your welfare. You may also wish to discuss things with your local association of disabled people to obtain further information on schemes of independent living, as well as the accommodation officer at your chosen place of study.

7.7 Obtain a breakdown of contents of your course

Having considered the challenges of gaining access to your place of study and living arrangements there, together with expenses, let us now suppose that you have been successful in gaining a place at the chosen establishment, and are ready to embark upon the course. Each course is likely to be taught through a set of lectures, and there will also be seminars and tutorials. There will be periods of assessment and examinations which could take a number of forms, including orals, practical tasks and written work. On top of all these, you will need time to relax, socialise or play sport. Thus the experience of post-school study could be considered as consisting of three things: the process of learning, the process of assessment and the process of unwinding and letting off steam. I now wish to examine each of these factors in a little more detail. My experience as an undergraduate student at Brunel was reading for a maths degree, and obviously different degrees may very well have a different mixture of the types of assessment or method of learning. An English degree, for example, may consist of far more written work in both coursework and examinations than a music or geography degree, which could have much more practical assignments. However, many of the ideas of successful learning and revision are common to most courses, be they A-levels, diplomas or degrees, and it is these ideas I wish to concentrate on now.

7.8 Lectures

The main way of collecting data, and storing it for future reference when you are assessed at a later date, is the lecture, where the aim is for you to sit in a class and listen to a teacher talking and explaining things, on which you are supposed to take notes. Lectures often last about 50 minutes each, with a short gap in between, and there will be several lectures each day, covering different topics and different sections of your course. Attending the vast majority of your lectures is very important throughout your course, because the work involved tends to get harder and more complex as time goes on and also often depends upon earlier results, and only a thorough understanding of these will enable you to make progress. There will no doubt be occasional times, such as when you are ill or have a pressing family emergency, when it may not be practical to attend a lecture, but even here you should contact the lecturer concerned and ask whether any notes on the work covered can be provided, or what action you can take to fill in the gap in what you are taught.

7.8a Before you even go to a lecture, plan ahead

Make sure you have all the necessary equipment with you such as pens, pencils, erasers, rulers and calculators. Do try to be prompt, as it can be very off-putting and distracting to a lecturer if they keep being interrupted by latecomers. By looking at your previous notes you may be able to visualise what the speaker will talk about (or they may have told the class in advance). If this is the case, you may want to try to investigate some of this material before the class. I have done this on many occasions throughout my BSc and found it very useful, as I already had an overall idea of the properties to be discussed and any remaining items I still had queries on were often answered for me during the lecture. For example, if I knew there was going to be a discussion on how to find the real roots of cubic equations, then I would already have found some textbooks on the subject and started them. Even just a flick through, learning just two or three points can help. It also gave me additional inner confidence knowing I was a step ahead of many of my peers!

On the other hand though, do not spend *too* long doing this. Be aware that you probably have plenty of other lectures and topics to consider as well, and should generally try to spend approximately an equal amount of time on each. If you find one particular section of your course more difficult, you might spend a little longer on it, but if you do this to an extreme it can be counter-productive. I once spent nearly all my time on one particular module I was finding especially testing, ended up doing well in it, but then badly underperfomed in many of the topics I was supposed to be good at as I had forgotten a lot of the work or missed new ideas. This forced my overall average mark down. Organising your workload is an important skill that can be acquired only through experience and if you are concerned in any way about your ability to do this effectively you should consult your personal tutor or the lecturers concerned.

7.8b Coping inside the lecture room

Once you arrive at the lecture room you should carefully consider where to sit. Resist the temptation to sit right at the back and natter to your best friend; it may seem more fun at the time writing jokes to one another in the margins when the lesson seems boring and difficult, but it will not do you any good in the long run! Every part of a lecture matters, and the parts that seem the toughest matter most. Many ideas on results, facts and formulae are interwoven with each other, and if you miss bits of information you are likely to have an incomplete picture of the situation under discussion, just like a man with one eye trying to view the landscape. It is often a good idea to sit towards the front of the lecture room, especially if you would otherwise have trouble reading any writing that the teacher is putting onto the blackboard or projector. It also helps to prevent people's heads getting in the way of your field of view. If you feel a bit vulnerable you may want to sit nearer the middle part of the room, but wherever you choose should be comfortable, not too hot or cold, and a position you feel you can concentrate in.

Next we have to think about methods of making notes once the lecturer actually starts talking. If you are very lucky, you may find that handouts of the work are provided, in which case most of the recording of information is already done for you. Otherwise you should be aware that many teachers speak quite quickly, even when they are expecting you to copy what they say word for word. If you are having trouble keeping up, remember that it is not always necessary to jot down every single thing, so long as you state the *key* points, or theorems, or methods and the like under discussion. If you have understood these, you can always fill in any gaps later, on little details such as grammar. Alternatively, if you are still concerned, you could ask the lecturer at the end of the lesson (it is not normally a good idea to interrupt while they are talking unless there is a clear opportunity of class dialogue with the teacher). Or, you might be able to obtain additional assistance from a non-medical support worker to sit in on some of your lectures and help take notes for you (contact the disability needs office at your place of study for further details on this), but make sure you can understand their notes!

7.8c *What to do after the lecture*

Once the lecture is over, it is a good idea to go over your notes anyway as soon as is practically possible, to make sure you can understand the main points. You may find it helpful to highlight or underline key words and phrases to make it easier to remember the ideas involved. You might also have question sheets handed out, and you should obviously try these. Sometimes it is difficult to be able to fit in *all* the questions when you have other demands and deadlines from other lecturers, but you could make a note of the points where you have got stuck so you can ask the teacher later. It is better to do a bit less and understand it totally rather than try to do everything in a rushed manner and not grasp important results. No one can expect to know all the work at once. You should be reviewing and revising work steadily throughout your course rather than panicking two weeks before the exams about how on earth you are going to cope. The brain can concentrate on something for only so long at any one time, so 'little and often' are the key words. Study a topic for about 40 minutes, take a ten-minute break for a cup of tea, then return refreshed for another 40 minutes of work. Any points or questions that you are stuck with can normally be discussed in the more informal setting of a seminar.

7.9 Seminars, workshops and tutorials

Here again the main aim is to learn more about the work but, unlike lectures, these periods are usually in a more relaxed atmosphere and provide a chance to ask questions on what was covered in the lectures in more detail than would be possible there. It also gives an opportunity to 'iron out' those parts of the topic covered that you found harder to follow or understand. Be ready for these times, and have with you a list of any queries you have. You may, of course, have to wait your turn while the other students attending ask questions themselves, but you should never be afraid to speak up and seek assistance. The mere fact that the set-up of these kinds of study periods can vary from week to week, depending on the topic under discussion and the number of people attending, can make them slightly unpredictable in a social sense, which might cause some anxiety to the autistic person, who can have difficulty picking up hints rapidly in the situation (are the other students asking queries individually to the lecturer, or is the lecturer asking questions as practice to see who among the students can put their hand up first with an answer?). If in doubt, ask the lecturer.

7.9a *The unpredictable elements of seminars, workshops and tutorials*

For most people, a request for you to stand up in front of the others for a couple of minutes to try to explain the solution to a question may seem innocent enough, especially if a couple of others have already done so and people are taking it in turns. But to someone with autism, being put on the spot like this, unprepared, could be very frightening, along with a number of other possibilities such as 'Please hand these sheets to Tony and Sara'. The autistic student may have trouble remembering names and not know what to say in this instance, fearing the others will laugh if he tells the truth that he has no idea who these two people are. You may have a one-to-one session with your tutor or lecturer (often called tutorials) and even in a seminar or workshop there are likely to be fewer people attending than in the lectures, since many lectures incorporate several groups of people studying 'overlapping' modules in their different courses (a maths-with-management student may study some common elements of his course with a maths-and-statistics student, with both students attending algebra and computing lectures). At the end of the day you can only deal with the less rigid structure of these forms of study by experiencing them often. They are an important way of aiding you to understand your work more thoroughly, and should not be regarded as a 'soft option' which you do not need to attend. It is up to you to make the most of them. Do not expect the lecturer to do your work for you in these periods either; rather, they should point you in the right direction so that you can attempt it and make progress. In motor-racing terms, understanding those parts of your work you did not before through discussing them in one of these small group situations could be compared to taking a pit-stop periodically, making sure that the wheels and other mechanical parts of the car are in good working order and that you are ready and refreshed to start the race again. If you miss your session and do not make sure you have a secure foundation, you may fail to grasp a key result which will be used in the next lecture and one of your wheels could come off round the next bend!

7.10 Examinations and assessments

7.10a *The importance of planning ahead*

The two-week examination period that is often operated at the end of each term or semester at college or university can be the most feared and nervy time for any student, and it can be especially so for the autistic one, who may underperform if feeling pressured or unwell. A thorough knowledge of most of the course material, obtained from having carefully revised notes, can mellow this level of anxiety a bit, but it is also a good idea to attempt past or trial exam papers beforehand. Many autistic students have quite good functional knowledge but are some-times put off by a different style or format of questions in the exams, or perhaps fail to grasp exactly what the questions are demanding of them. Even in mathematics, the words 'show' and 'prove' a property or theorem might sound similar requests, yet 'prove' is more demanding and requires vigorous intervention, whereas 'show' needs only a demonstration that a statement is true. I have found through my own experience that where initially you need enough basic know-how to make progress in your course, there is no substitute to attempting mock exams in this way to improve your knowledge and style of presentation. You will get to familiarise yourself with certain key phrases or words and have a better understanding of what is required with each question, as well as an idea of how well you are keeping track of the time.

Many of the recommendations for surviving the actual exams are common sense. Find out in good time exactly where and when each exam is. Get all the necessary equipment ready the night before (pens, rulers, erasers, etc.). The last thing you want is to arrive late and in a state because you could not find your essentials or did not know where the exam room was. If you are worried about oversleeping you may wish to get a friend to give you a wake-up call to put your mind at rest (in case your alarm clock does not go off or you do not have an alarm clock, for example). Try to get a good night's sleep, although this may be easier said than done. Certainly do not go clubbing at the disco until 2 a.m. the night before. If you have a calculator you should check if you are allowed to take it into the exam room; sometimes only a certain kind is permitted and sometimes they may be banned altogether. Once inside, listen very carefully to any instructions from the invigilators, and when allowed, read the directions on the papers very carefully. Pay particular attention to the number of questions in each section of the exam you must attempt, and if you have a choice of questions, glance through the whole of each question – many of them may start off with easier parts and then get progressively more difficult. Starting with the questions you feel most confident with is often a good rule of thumb. It will give you confidence and the knowledge that you have probably already obtained most of the marks for them before you go on to other perhaps more tricky-looking ones. Once in a statistics exam where I had to answer three questions I noticed that one of them was exactly on what I had been revising the previous day. I immediately worked through it knowing that I had accumulated roughly a third of the total marks available in about the first 20 minutes. Remember to keep an eye on the time too, and attempt to spend roughly an equal amount of minutes on each of those questions worth equal marks.

7.10b Don't be thrown off guard by little details

It will often be little details about the exams that throw you off guard or distract you. Even such things as where to write your candidate number or position number, or being able to tie your exam papers together with string can prove significantly worrying – in extreme cases (it happened to me!) I worried more about not being able to do these things than answering the main questions. If you are at all rattled, just raise your hand and wait until you get the attention of one of the investigators in charge. *Never attempt to cheat in any way,* by using hidden notes, copying someone else's work, or trying any other method. You are likely to be caught out and could be disqualified completely from the exam or from your course. If, after trying your best in an exam, you still underperform and do not get the marks you hope for – fair enough – you can learn from the experience for next time. But any attempt not to play fair is something you will have to live with for the rest of your life and could tarnish your reputation and opportunities in everything you do, and nothing is worth letting that happen.

7.10c Organise your workload

You may have several modules of study within your course that are assessed with continuous assignments, either partially (say 20% of the total marks) or (less frequently) in its entirety. Coursework tasks obviously do not have the intense time restrictions (a few hours at most) that the written examinations do, and in that sense this can reduce anxiety levels, but you will still normally have deadlines to adhere to. Be sensible and allow enough time to complete these, or at least have a good attempt at them. Those individuals leaving everything until the night before will almost certainly not finish or end up rushing the work and losing marks because of careless mistakes. You may also have a separate individual project (an extended piece of work where you will normally be assisted by a member of staff), particularly in your final year. You will be able to talk about any such project with your personal tutor as well as your allocated teacher (if not the same). All this may seem like incredibly hard work, and it is. No one undergoing a higher education course should be under any illusion about this. You will probably be stretched harder than ever before into understanding very complex and detailed work and problem-solving. But the rewards at the end can be greater than anything you have experienced before as well! That proud moment of picking up your award, or perhaps shaking hands with the Chancellor at the graduation ceremony, wearing your mortar board and gown, is one to treasure for ever, as well as a qualification that most people can only envy. Although remember you may still need help with the little things, such as putting the outfit and the mortar board on the right way round (I did!).

7.11 Extra challenges at postgraduate level

At the top end of the ability range, a very few of you might be studying for a degree, or even several degrees. When you first start attending university it will normally be for a first degree which if successful will allow you to put initials after your name, such as a BSc (Bachelor of Science) or a BA (Bachelor of Arts). Many degrees are three years in length, but can be four years if work placements are included as part of the course. Even a first degree will demand an understanding at a very high level for you to be successful.

If individuals have performed well enough in their first degree (usually with a first or upper second class honours mark) they will have the option of pursuing their studies with a second, 'higher', degree, leading to a Master's degree or a doctorate/PhD. There could be a number of additional challenges facing autistic people undertaking such a feat. First there is the fact that the types of financial support and help mentioned earlier in this chapter for first degrees and lower courses tend to be more restricted in this instance, as the government seems more reluctant to fund people in the minority. And if you are seriously considering postgraduate study you will be in the minority – of those élite people with a chance to be amongst the best in the world academically!

The other chief difficulty that can arise with a higher degree is its often 'lack of rigid timetable' content of work in the course. There may have been a certain comfort for the autistic individual in undergraduate work in that while demanding, it often involved attending lectures and seminars at the same time each week with an orderly routine to get used to. There may have been assignments, or even project work, where one was made to work independently at times, but usually this constituted only a small part of the overall course being followed. In sharp contrast, postgraduate students have to organise their own study time for almost the whole duration of their work, especially if they are following a research degree (such as a Master's or PhD) rather than a 'taught' Master's, although they may attend some lectures in all cases in the early part of their course for preliminary understanding of the basics of their field of study. The students arrange periodic meetings with their supervisor to discuss progress, which may vary from week to week according to how their research develops. This lack of organised structure is unfortunately precisely the kind of set-up that can prove unsettling and stressful to someone with autism, and once again regular support and advice from tutors, disability teams and social services can prove vital to continued progress.

Most postgraduate students are then required to write and type up a 'thesis' (a precise account of their work and how they have used their knowledge of the subject-matter to solve complex problems and draw conclusions). Such work can be hundreds of pages long and requires a high level of self-discipline and deter-mination to complete it. Many of the comforts of a first-degree support in an emotional sense may not be present here. You might have had one or two good friends who encouraged you or helped you out in instances where they attended the same lectures as you, and there would always be other academic staff who could probably help you with problems in your work. But most of the material covered at postgraduate level is highly specialised and the chances are that if you cannot get hold of your supervisor, you could find it very difficult to find others who understand enough about what you are studying to be able to help you. In addition, very often the editing and eliminating mistakes procedure neces-sary to obtain a final version of your thesis acceptable to be examined will take almost as long as the main research and pro-duction of the initial copy of your work. Many degrees of this nature also require you to undergo an oral exam at the end, where you will have to stand up in front of a panel of teachers trained in your speciality, and discuss your work and the results and conclusions that you were able to reach from it. They will probably ask you questions about it as well. This procedure requires several 'mock' attempts (with your supervisor, say) and practice in giving a talk, and can demand nerves of steel. You then will be awarded your degree if they are satisfied with your oral presentation and your thesis is up to the required standard. All these points may sound very negative, but I am a firm believer that if someone wants something badly enough they will find a way to manage and cope, and rise to the challenge. I have been through the whole experience. At times when I undertook my postgraduate degree in maths, it seemed as if I was climbing Mount Everest at a snail's pace. But step by step I climbed up, and eventually reached my goal in graduation at the summit. And showed the world I meant business. And that being autistic does not have to limit your goals or achievements one bit. The potential to become world-beaters is in all of us. It just has to be unlocked in the right way, through correct help, organisational skills to a high intensity, and sheer will-power.

7.12 Relaxation – give yourself time to unwind

No matter how intense your course demands are, it is also important to give your body enough rest and time to unwind from the stresses of all those assignments and deadlines. Most establishments will have a social club (such as a student union) which organises social activities, and if you are the sporty type there will usually be loads of different sports to try your hand at, from football to table tennis, or perhaps even something more exotic like rock-climbing. Obviously you could feel very shy about the prospect of starting new activities for the first time, as it will involve meeting new people – one of the things we find difficult by definition of our disability – so you may wish to go with someone at first, perhaps with a support worker. Even if you feel you are too tired with all the course work or do not have time to become the new superstar of your establishment's sports club, it is

116 SURVIVAL STRATEGIES FOR THE AUTISM SPECTRUM

still important to give yourself a little time to yourself. Even an hour a day, perhaps before you go to bed, maybe watching a TV programme, can help get yourself into a more relaxed state and a better frame of mind for the next day. There is also the option of trying a number of relaxation exercises or massages to help ease muscle tension. Much of the information on recreation and leisure activities can be found in the library or sports building of your place of study.

7.13 Learn from experiences

Your years spent in higher education can turn out to be the most fulfilling and confidence-building time of your life. You just need to be organised and have a real desire to succeed. Remember that there are many helping hands to ask help from, in addition to your normal care manager, tutor and disability officer. These include counsellors, other lecturers, medical-centre staff and the like. Information on assignments and examination techniques will normally be available in your place of study's library, or ask one of the lecturers or your personal tutor. Inevitably, there will sometimes be things that crop up unexpectedly and can prove worrisome. These are often the sort of practical tasks that most others would not expect you to be anxious about if they were not aware of your condition, such as putting your tie on the right way round, or helping to distribute a booklet round the class to a selection of students and not being able to pick out the correct ones who require it. I would say that anyone who experiences this sort of thing can learn from it, since it is a fact that we can learn more from our mistakes than from what we find easy. Strategies can then be drawn up to handle the events better next time round – for example, practise doing your tie up under supervision on several occasions until you get more confident with it, or jot down the names of some of your fellow students and ask them to put their hands up if they require these leaflets. I shall be concentrating more on the unpredictable nature of occurrences and their effects on autistic people in Chapter 10, but generally you should always try to communicate with someone for advice if something is really troubling you, no matter how trivial it might seem. Once we are feeling better or are reassured, we tend to work better too and make greater progress in our studies.

CHAPTER 8

The World of Sport as an Aid

In this chapter, I shall be taking a closer look at the role that participating in sport can have on helping autistic people with their social and physical development. The demands and challenges of taking part in an activity can teach us a lot about our physical and mental strengths, and also require good communication skills in relating to other people – vital in the progress of your social 'know-how' – while the rewards of doing well can give a sense of satisfaction and intense pride. You may remember, for example, your family trying tennis or hockey once or twice in the long summer months, but all too often this may take place on an overgrown court without a proper net, and then perhaps two weeks later something else of interest occurred, making you forget the activity and move on. To make real progress, it is usually far better to join a local club of the sport of your choice. You will be assessed in your standard and will be able to meet and play with others of similar ability to your own. You will also get more opportunity to play on a regular basis and will be given advice on outfits, equipment (rackets, balls and so on) and etiquette.

8.1 Equipment and clothing

When a soldier goes into battle, he will feel ready to do so only when he is well protected with a good uniform and means of protecting himself. In a similar vein, it is very important for one to plan ahead for a contest in sport, long before you reach the venue. Your clothes must be ones that you feel comfortable in to play and run about, and they will also depend on which sport you are playing, the weather (for outdoor pursuits) and perhaps the importance of the contest. Sometimes your choice of outfit just requires a certain amount of common sense for instance. In hot summer weather, most people playing outside prefer to wear white or light-coloured clothes that tend to reflect the heat rather than absorb it. In colder weather, we should wrap up warm. Be aware that sometimes even in the summer it can become much colder later on, or after sunset, so it is a good idea to have an extra jumper or jacket with you in case you need it. Conversely, even with indoor activities such as table tennis, many private clubs have certain dress codes to be followed (you will find this out when you join).

For most sports (unless you choose something exotic like scuba diving!) your shoes can be the most important part of your outfit, and it is vital that they feel comfortable – too small and they can rub on your feet causing blisters, too big and they may make you trip over. It is often necessary to 'wear in' a new pair of trainers to get used to them (wear them perhaps for a couple of hours inside your home several times first). Remember that the most expensive trainers are not necessarily the most comfortable, and complications arise when one of your feet is bigger than the other. You can decide only by trying on different ones and seeking advice from the shop you are purchasing from. Make sure you know your shoe size (10, 11, 12, etc.) because you will be asked for it. Even the best-fitted trainers may feel strange for the first day or so until your feet become accustomed to them. This can apply to other items of clothing too. Do take dress precautions seriously. Resist the temptation to use that mouldy old pair of trainers with holes in the bottom or that pair of trousers that feel too tight and restrict movement. By dressing appropriately, you will not only have more fun and feel more at ease but also reduce the risk of injury (through falling over for example).

8.2 So how much will it all cost?

When you are planning your participation in your chosen sport, you must carefully consider the cost of both the membership of any club involved and also the equipment required. Many clubs offer different types of membership at different rates, for example on a yearly or monthly basis, or perhaps a day membership at a cheaper rate where you can only play between 10 a.m. and 4 p.m. In addition, you may be able to obtain discounts because of your disability and circumstances (you would need proof of this though, so if not certain check with your advisers/carers). You must weigh up the type of membership that will be of the best practical use to you, given the restrictions of your income. With equipment also it is important to get a fine balance between spending too much for a professional piece of equipment that is not really required when you are starting out, and not paying enough and using unsuitable items. For instance, for playing racket sports such as tennis and squash, there is an enormous (and bewildering for many!) variety of different rackets on sale in the shops, with different sizes, tensions (in the strings) and material used. These often 'fine' details are important for a high-level per-former who may want to vary the spin they impart on the ball or to generate more power on their serve. But for a starter, it is not necessary to spend £200 on an 'expert' racket, so long as it feels comfortable (not too heavy) with a suitable handle for gripping.

8.3 Making a game plan

Returning for a moment to our soldier going into battle, we realise that he will not want to do so without a detailed plan of action on how to proceed. He would wish to have some idea of the opposition's strengths and weaknesses and what action they may take in response to him. Our soldier will be putting his wits and strategy on the line against the enemy and trying to stay a step ahead of them, by anticipating their moves before they can make them. He will also be aware that conflict can be unpredictable so will wish to have a back-up plan in case things do not work out as he expected. The number of options available to you in terms of different game plans will depend on a number of factors such as the sport concerned, how good a player you are, and your standard and type of opponent. Let us consider some different situations:

8.3a Case 1: When you have just one opponent

This could be when you are undertaking a singles match in a racket sport, such as squash or tennis. Even a fairly simple mastery of the basic shots of the game (such as service, forehand and backhand) can be used to improve your chances. If you always hit the ball close to your opponent or to her strengths, it follows that it will be easier for her to send the ball back to you. So try to find her weaknesses and exploit them! Most (although not all) players tend to be stronger on their forehand side than on the backhand, so why not aim more returns at her backhand side? But do throw in the occasional forehand shot as well, because if you *always* hit the returns to her backhand it will become too predictable. Another plan would be to try and hit the ball as far away from your opponent as you can with each return, to try to tire her out with all that running after the ball. If you have previous knowledge of your opponent's style of play, or get a chance to watch her play someone else first, you could make notes on which shots she appears to be more successful with and which strokes she finds difficult, and then formulate how you could try to outwit her by playing mainly to her weaker points.

8.3b Case 2: When you have two opponents

There are many occasions at club level when people play in a team of four (two against two) in racket sports. Indeed with a sport such as tennis it is actually more common to play in this way. Unfortunately for someone with autism, this situation can become considerably harder than playing one against one, because now not only do we have two opponents who will no doubt possess different strengths and weaknesses, but we also have a partner player to consider. It is often necessary to communicate rapidly with your partner as to who will take the next shot for instance, by shouting 'mine!' or 'yours!' and when to run out the way to avoid crashing into your partner! The social 'know-how' to do this is often lacking with an autistic individual and, unless the partner has been made aware beforehand of these possible discrepancies, frustration can quickly build. I would therefore suggest that until you are very confident you choose a partner who is aware of and sympathetic to your condition, and you discuss with them beforehand how you will deal with any situations that require rapid communicational skills between you, along with a basic (but sound) strategy for your overall gameplan, e.g. let us both keep our returns low as our opponents both love smashing high balls for a winner.

8.3c Case 3: When you have many opponents

There are some sports, such as football, where you will be facing a large number of opponents but also people playing on your side. The basic idea here is to work as a team, with individual players doing their best to help the others on their side. In one way, this can produce the most challenging scenario of all for someone with autism, as they will have to be aware of who is on 'their' side and who is not, as well as the often unspoken rules of the game and exactly what is expected of them. Different players on any one team often have different duties, such as an attacking player in football who tries to score goals could be the role for one, whereas another could be a defender who tries to keep the opposition from scoring rather than trying to score themselves. A team could be thought of as a chain which we hope holds together, but any underperformance from one individual can lead to a break in that chain, disrupting the intended structure and plan of attack. In these situations, the overall coach is the best person to discuss with on how to play. You must have a clear understanding before the game of exactly what role you are expected to play within your team, and also how to cope with any potentially challenging social occurrences.

8.3d Case 4: No direct opponents

There are also sports, such as golf, where you are obviously still pitted against others in terms of a scoresheet, but it is entirely in your hands how well you do individually. Although the good or bad performance of others on the field will be out of your control in cases like these, you can still discuss with your coach or teacher and produce a plan on what shots to attempt to try to maximise yourself doing well. And while it can take a lot of patience, things like golf can be practised on your own for as long as you wish before you consider competitive play.

8.3e Case 5: What if your gameplan is not working?

Have at least one back-up plan

The mere fact that matches can be unpredictable requires us to plan ahead in case our initial strategy does not work as well as we had hoped. Perhaps our opponent in tennis is much better with her backhand now than we realised and we need to hit more returns to her forehand, or perhaps our opposing team in football has used an unexpected attacking formation to threaten our goal and we need to change our team's approach to the match in the second half. By looking ahead and producing these plans for action before the contest, we can be ready with a simple instruction to proceed to the different style of play which could make all the difference and win us that vital match. Not having any prede-termined plan of action could be like our soldier stepping onto the battlefield blindfolded, having no idea what to do and being vulnerable to attack.

8.4 Fitness and stamina

8.4a Getting started

The other important consideration to bear in mind before taking part in a sporting contest is that of our state of fitness and physical readiness. For many people the idea of a game of, say, squash or tennis is just that, even if they have been lying on the sofa all morning watching television. They will then rush straight onto court and proceed to whack the ball at one another in a haphazard way, with no real plan of what shots to play. But stop to think for a moment, and you will soon realise that this is not the best way to proceed. If you owned an old car that had not been used for several weeks, you would not expect to drive it at 70 mph straight away. Instead, you would need to let the engine warm up, and accelerate gradually. In the same way, our bodies need time to warm up after a period of inactivity. Many sports impose great demands on your muscles and working parts of your feet, hands and body, and if you are not fully warmed up, you stand much more risk of pulling a muscle or incurring an injury. On the other end of the scale there are those people who are super-fit and spend nearly all their time in the gym. This may be expected if they are world-class sportsmen, but for the average club player a compromise between these two extremes is advisable. Even just five or ten minutes warming up can make all the difference and get you in a much better state to play, so resist the temptation not to bother because you have not got time or it seems boring.

8.4b Types of exercise

There are many kinds of warm-up exercises to choose from, and these will depend partly on the kind and level of participation of your particular sport, one of the simplest being to simply run around a playing field or tennis court two or three times. Others include standing on your toes, moving your arms and wrists in circular motions, and turning your head and shoulders. Just a minute or so spent on each main part of the body will soon have you ready to go. If your level of participation is high enough to have a coach, they will be able to provide you with the advice you need on an appropriate set of warm-up exercises. Otherwise you can refer to appropriate guide books, and check with an adult or carer that you have a proper understanding of how to go about the exercises. Remember also that it is often a good idea to do some brief warm-down exercises as well. Most people forget about this, but if you do, after you have been playing intensely for several hours, it may be like that car driver doing 70 mph and then trying to stop immediately. You may feel fine at the start of play, but in a long contest you can very quickly become tired. For outdoor pursuits, make sure you have plenty of liquids with you to drink, especially on a hot day (make sure these are appropriate liquids too, not too many fizzy drinks for example!). Equally, be especially careful in wet or cold weather – rain or hidden ice can make that football field or tennis court quite a dangerous slippery place. If in doubt, do not risk it; play next time or go elsewhere.

8.4c Types of injury

If you have not been very active in a sport beforehand, it may be a good idea to talk to your coach (or doctor) about any precautions to take to avoid injury, especially if you have any symptoms that can restrict your movement or you would be liable to injury with any sudden jolt or movement. Even allowing for good warm-up exercises, even professional world-class sports players can be affected by a number of injuries. One example of such an injury is known as 'tennis elbow', which involves discomfort in the arm or wrist that a tennis player holds his racket with, as a result of overuse of muscles. There are often regarded to be two levels of injury: one that causes mild discomfort but allows you to play on (such as a corn on the foot) and the other that can cause severe discomfort (like a pulled muscle). I once pulled a muscle but tried to play on to the end of what seemed like an important point in a tennis match, but was then in great pain for two weeks and could hardly move about at all. I would advise that you avoid the same mistake and wherever something is clearly hampering your movement you should always proceed on the side of caution and get it treated or at least rested before continuing play. It is not worth risking your long-term health, no matter what the position in a game or match.

8.5 Techniques and execution of shots

We have spent some time considering pre-match preparation, but now let us turn our attention to the situation of actually being at the arena and participating in your sport. Much is said about the so-called technique of a player, how the weight of your body and its position should change the type of shots you play, but it is important not to get bogged down by a minefield of different information. The golden rule initially is to keep things simple and not expect instant miracles, because there are all sort of traps lying in wait for an autistic individual who takes everything literally, even from notes in an instruction manual. One needs to be aware that there are certain things that may not be discovered until later on and might not even be noticed in a coaching session. I will now examine one such example of this which can happen to those four per cent or so individuals of the population who happen to be left-handed (such as me) and have to live in a world where the vast majority of the population are right-handed. This can lead us left-handers to feel the odd one out at times, just like having autism.

8.6 A trap for the unwary left-hander

The following misadventure happened to me while playing tennis, but it could easily happen to other autistic individuals in most racket sports if they are caught unaware. I had been playing the game a number of months and thought I was starting to improve. One day, an adult I knew had been watching me play, and instead of praising me, he remarked, 'I thought you were becoming a good tennis player, so how come you are playing all your shots inside out, and your grip is back to front?' At the time I was rather upset and perplexed to hear this, as I had carefully studied an instruction book on tennis grips and how to hold a racket while playing the standard shots such as the forehand and backhand. And I had followed those instructions precisely as they had been stated. A bit later on, it dawned on me. Instructions from tennis books and coaches on how to grip the racket or position the body and arms while playing a shot are normally given on the basis of the learner being right-handed, simply because the majority of people are. Unfortunately, this is usually not specifically stated, just assumed, and I had not been aware that commands such as 'rotate your grip 45° anti-clockwise' actually implied 45° *clockwise* for a left-hander, and so consequently I ended up doing things back to front. So remember to think in the reverse sense if you are left-handed (e.g. a shot played on your left will be a forehand to you, but a backhand to a right-handed person).

8.7 Advantages of correct technique

Having a sound technique while executing a shot in sport could be compared to driving a car in which all of the main parts such as the engine and tyres are in good working order while actually moving. A good grip on the road will reduce the risk of skidding, while having a healthy engine and plenty of fuel will reduce the possibility of breakdown. Similarly, knowing how to go about producing consistent returns in a racket sport, say, without errors, will enable you to put your opponent under pressure to make a mistake herself, and at the same time reduce the pressure on you and increase your chance of being successful in the long run. Besides, in many participation sports such as table tennis it is actually not allowed to hit many shots such as the serve in certain ways, and you may find yourself being penalised and having a point deducted without realising why unless you already know the techniques allowed! There can also be times, even when things are going wrong, that *making* them go wrong in the correct way, using the proper technique, can save you from getting injured or being disqualified. For instance, if a champion down-hill skier falls off his skis halfway down a mountain, knowing how to land and roll over to cushion himself could make a critical difference to how badly he hurts himself. In the same way a gymnastics enthusiast falling off the beam from a somersault should know how to fall and an ice skater must know, should he fall, how to recover and get up again quickly before he loses more points on the all important scoreboard.

8.8 Adjust your choice of shot according to the position of a contest

As well as trying to exploit your opponent's weaknesses, you also have to consider how reliable your own shots are. The shot you choose to use could be affected by the probability of it being successful, and by the game score. If you are match-point down, for example in a tennis match, you *have* to win the next point to stay in the match, so you would be unlikely to opt to play a volley if you feel very unconfident with volleys and only get one out of six in the court. You would instead choose another shot, like a forehand that has more chance of getting the ball back into play, at the expense of aggression. On the other hand, if the score is in your favour, perhaps three match-points to you, it might be worth risking an ambitious smash or outright winner. It could win you the match and even if it does not, you will still have another two chances to do so.

8.9 The mental side of sport and sporting etiquette

8.9a Effort produced is more important than external wins and losses

In every singles match of a knockout tournament in sport, one player must end up the winner, the other the loser. The key element is to take part and enjoy your chosen sport. It follows that we should care about whether we win or not, and should try to do everything within our ability and the written rules to try to do so, but the eventual outcome may depend on a number of factors beyond our control. Perhaps a stroke of luck on a call helped your opponent to win a crucial point, or a freak gust of wind affected your concentration, forcing you to make an uncharacteristic error in executing a shot, which resulted in the score changing significantly in your opponent's favour. In order to improve one's standards and become a better player in one's chosen sport, it is necessary to play different opponents so that experience can be formed of many different situations, and during this process people must realise that there will be many times when they will lose a contest. In a singles tournament of 64 individuals, 63 of them will be losers at some stage, and only one will be the winner. It is important to approach this fact in the right way. We cannot dwell too much on external scores, twists of fate or other factors beyond our control. What we can do, however, is to ensure that we put the maximum effort into each point. If this is done, you have nothing to be ashamed of. In fact, the individual who handles losing better will not only be respected more by his opponents, but is also more likely to learn through the experience and become a better player next time around.

8.9b Win with modesty, lose graciously

First, you will never know the final outcome of a match until the last point has been played. Even if you are three match-points up, you cannot assume that you will definitely win. Your opponent could stage a comeback himself. You should acknowledge the fact that this happens, and when you lose a match, it is almost always because your opponent has just been better on the day. Being mentally tough after a heavy loss takes guts, especially if you have been stretching yourself to the limit to try to win. But it will not help to make excuses such as 'It was too sunny' or 'I wasn't feeling well'. You will make things easier for yourself and your opponent by being strong enough not to complain. Equally, if you win, try to be tactful and considerate to the loser. After all, you know what it feels like to be in their position. Avoid careless remarks such as, 'Beat you! I'm better than you now. You never stood a chance!' Instead you could say, 'Well played' or 'Hard luck' as you shake hands, or, 'We both played well, that was a great match'. By keeping control of your emotions, you can enjoy the elation of a win without going over the top. Equally, you can take the disappointment of a loss in your stride and not get too despondent.

8.9c Be fair and stick to the rules

Whatever your chosen sport, it is very important to play fair at all times and abide by the rules. For instance, with racket sports, there will occur a number of tight calls during a match where the ball can land very close to the edge of the court – you should always be honest on such calls. Resist the temptation to call a close ball out on a crucial point when you have seen it touch the line. After all, put yourself in the reverse situation – you would not like your opponent to dish out that sort of treatment to you. Often, if neither of you is sure about a tight call, or have a difference of opinion, the best thing to do is to call a 'let' which means you start again and the point is replayed. Another complication can occur when the score is forgotten (usually when your match is not being umpired!), so it is a good idea to state the score regularly to avoid arguments. Otherwise you could start again at a level score.

8.9d Never give up

It could be argued that the most counter-productive moments in a sporting contest mentally can come in the time between executing the shots, because it is here that the mind can wander. Suppose in a game of football you have just committed a careless foul which has resulted in a penalty being awarded to the opposition, resulting in them scoring a goal. It will be very tempting for you to then think 'How could I be so terrible? I may as well not bother with trying any more as there are only 15 minutes left so we will probably lose anyway'. This sort of thinking can only be counter-productive; indeed the very sight of you drooping your head and looking despondent will give people in your opposing team more confidence that they have the better of you, and make them more likely to score another goal! On the other hand, a bit of extra determination at this point could see you develop an opportunity for your team to score an equaliser. Not only will this have levelled the score, but it could demoralise the opposition, knowing that they had the lead and lost it. This could make your team more likely to score again and win the match. So try not to think ahead, or dwell on what has already happened, but *play for the moment*, and give your best effort throughout. Remember that matches like these have changed in the last few seconds of the game.

8.9e Help your partners

In many contests you must remember your partners as well as your opposition and rules of the game. Your partners will like to be praised now and then, so why not do so with a comment such as 'good shot' or 'well played' when they have won a good point. Not too often though – remember that you are not the commentary team for the match! Equally, it will not help to criticise your partners too much if they make a losing shot. They will no doubt be only too aware of how bad it might have looked without you reminding them. So be positive instead – why not comment 'better luck next time!'?

8.10 A word on different standards

In a sporting contest there will generally be three types of standard you will face.

8.10a Your opposition is considerably weaker than you

You can usually win the contest here fairly comfortably. This may seem easy, but remember that you are less likely to make progress towards becoming a better player when you can always win easily. In these cases you can either restrict yourself to playing only shots that you find more difficult or handicap yourself by giving them a head start in the scoring, to make it more challenging for you and fairer on your opponents.

8.10b Your opposition is roughly the same standard as you

This is perhaps the best situation to be in, with two equally opposing teams trying to outwit one another. In particular, if your opposition is marginally better than you and has often beaten you narrowly in the past, you have a great opportunity to improve your shot selection and match determination as you strive to finally outsmart your opponents.

8.10c Your opposition is considerably stronger than you

This can still be productive, provided you approach it in the right way: as a learning process that will eventually help your own game. Do not worry too much about the fact that you get walloped 6–0 in football, or 6–0, 6–1 in a tennis match. Instead make a note of details, like the type of tactics and shots that your opposition was using that won them the points and the match. Were they outrunning you? Maybe there were some faster and fitter footie players than you? Did you get aced off the tennis court by a more powerful service? Or perhaps your opposition just had better court sense and was able to catch you out of position with a set of passing shots? Whatever the reasons, it gives you an opportunity to review what aspects of your own game you need to work on in the next practice session.

8.11 What makes a champion?

We must at all times get things into perspective. A game in sport is just that – a game. You are not playing with your life at stake. We cannot all expect to be brilliant players like Boris Becker or Wayne Rooney, hitting winning shots all the time straight away. Learning to play a sport well is like any other learning process where we collect data in our minds through our experiences, so that we can apply that knowledge next time we are in a similar situation. Having a coach can certainly help steer us in the right direction to becoming an expert, but no amount of coaching can make a champion. Instead, the final thrust and determination has to come from the individual concerned. It comes with a person's total belief in their ability to do things well, the knowledge of how to out-think opponents and be one or even two or three steps ahead of them in the mind. Watch a good player hit a marvellous shot in a contest and note that they will not stand around for too long afterwards admiring it, but will already be moving and preparing in anticipation for their opposition's next move. They will also be able to assess the development of the match as it goes on, and make adjustments to their style of play if necessary to exploit the opposition's weaknesses to the full, as well as getting a good balance between playing too aggressively and too cautiously.

It is often necessary for an inspiring hopeful to alter a certain feature of their game under the watchful eye of their coach. This could be, for example, to change their type of grip in a racket sport to allow for greater speed or imparting of spin on the ball. Initially, there will be a period where this could be very difficult, as for a while until one gets used to the new type of shot there will be a period where one's performance appears to get worse. The temptation when put under pressure in, say, a match situation, is to revert to the original grip that one felt more familiar with in the past, but it is a temptation which must be resisted in order to make real progress, as putting up with short-term difficulties can mean long and far-reaching extra successes further down the line. A true champion is one who has the variety of different shots perfected which are necessary to being able to beat and counter the challenge of a large number of opponents, by using and being able to produce the right shots required on the day for each opposition.

Especially at a high level of performance, a sportsperson will know that that their welfare and success can never be guaranteed. One day you could be the national hero having won the Open in golf or the Championship at Wimbledon, or in the winning team of the football World Cup, then a bad bounce of a ball or a twisted ankle could make you the villain who missed that vital penalty to get us knocked out of the World Cup. Do not be under any illusion – the public is not generally sympathetic to an under-perfomance, be it someone with autism or not. For every success story of a champion there will be countless others who failed to make the grade, by an unforeseen injury, a cruel twist of fate or letting nerves get to them. However, let us not be too negative, there is no reason why you cannot make the breakthrough into the top élite, providing you are prepared to put in the large amount of preparation, work and training required and have the determination and belief to keep going when things get tough.

8.12 Coaching others yourself

Finally I round off this chapter by examining one of the most challenging things that an autistic person can attempt, namely to coach others in their chosen sport. Even for the average person, coaching others is not easy. It requires not only a thorough understanding of the rules of the game, but also an ability to communicate your knowledge to the learners in a way they will understand. For someone with autism, this latter fact can be especially demanding, perhaps even more so than simply participating in a team game, since here you must be aware of every other member in terms of being responsible for their welfare during the lesson. We cannot expect learners to make progress too quickly, just like a pupil studying for their GCSE exams could not be suddenly placed in a degree level assignment and be expected to cope. Just because a shot seems easy to us does not mean it will be to the others (imagine what it was like when you first learnt that shot). Coaching properly also needs an ability to judge how many instructions to give at once. It is possible to 'overcoach', giving your audience such a large number of commands such as grip, foot and body positions and movement that they can simply become overloaded and 'seize up' so to speak, unable to do anything productive. On the other hand, you must set a certain level of order in the class to avoid a complete lack of attention and no one listening to you at all. An experienced coach will be able to get a good balance between these two extremes.

For many years I have been a keen tennis player and watcher, and I am fascinated by the mental game as well as the more physical aspects of the sport. I have also become a patron of the Horizons Sports Club, where I assist the coaches in a series of tennis classes (based at the Bucks Indoor Tennis Centre in High Wycombe) which are aimed at providing crucial opportunities for the youngsters to develop their social interactions skills in a related and caring environment. The club is for disabled children aged between 5 and 12 who attend specialist schools locally, and caters for many other disabilities as well as autism. These include dyslexia, dyspraxia and cerebral palsy. It also provides sports such as swimming and indoor athletics for many others. One of my greatest joys of working in these classes is to see the intense happiness often expressed on the children's faces, almost as if all the worries of their world are taken away for these few moments of tranquillity, playing a sport that they love in an environment they feel safe in. It is as is someone has opened a window on their often lonely frustrating world, and they can come out for some fresh air and relief.

CHAPTER 9

The Challenge of Sharing Ideas with the Wider Audience

Learning how to live and cope with independence is not just a vital skill in its own right for autistic individuals, it also gives them an opportunity to help perhaps thousands or even millions of other people in similar positions to live more fulfilling lives. We can spread awareness of our own experiences in a variety of ways: as a presentation in a class, assembly, social skills group or, more ambitiously, in lectures, social functions, public speeches, television and radio. We can do it in written form in magazine and newspaper articles and books, electronically on computers and the Internet. In this chapter, I shall be examining the main points that enable an individual to communicate experiences and 'messages' to the outside world effectively. There are always ways of getting points across to people using perhaps unconventional methods, and I discuss those in more detail here.

9.1 Communication: preparations before the presentation

9.1a Look the part

Your 'presentation' of yourself when giving a talk should start before you even get to the place concerned. Remember, impressions count, so do make the effort to dress appropriately. Even if it is only a very informal meeting, you will still look better in a smart casual outfit rather than those old jeans full of holes. Put yourself in the reverse situation. If someone came to you to give a talk you would probably have a better opinion of them if they wore a smart set of clothes rather than looking scruffy. For longer presentations and more formal occasions a proper suit is advisable, perhaps with a tie and neat shirt as well. Be sensible. If you are not sure what is the best way to dress for an event, then ask the organiser or a good friend. And do not forget to make sure you can put the clothes on properly as well, because many autistic people can find this difficult. There is no point in buying a brilliant £200 suit, only to go into your presentation with your shirt hanging out, your tie on back to front and the collar not folded down properly. In addition, a well-dressed individual will look professional and show that he cares enough about his presentation to want to look good. Usually, at school, a uniform will be the expected dress.

9.1b Making notes

You will, of course, unless you are very confident (more on this later), be required to plan your presentation, and your approach to this is important for a successful outcome. Your notes and other reminders should be clear enough for you to understand what they mean and should contain the key points and overall framework of the presentation, but putting down every single point in detail can result in finding yourself hopelessly lost in a wad of material. So you must get a good happy medium between not making enough notes and making an excessive amount – this is especially important with longer presentations. For example, suppose you were asked to talk for a few minutes to a group of people to enlighten them as to what the main difficulties experienced by an individual with autism are. There is a multitude of different topics you could mention, but instead of writing a lengthy essay you could divide your talk into sections as follows (the personal experiences included are of course hypothetical ones – you will have to think up your own). These are some ideas you could use in any form of presentation.

Main difficulties (autism)

1. Normal social dialogue hard to grasp

(a) *Taking things literally* – my experience of 'eat my hat'.

(b) *Sarcasm* – my experience – person said 'lovely weather' when pouring with rain. When do people mean what they say?

2. Not knowing acceptable behaviour in front of others

(a) My experience – pretending to be *robotic*.

(b) My experience – individual called out '*be very quick please*' in queue.

(c) Asking someone's *age* not appropriate – my experience when I did.

(d) *Ignoring* people – e.g. if I had change for £10 note. I was frightened by a tall burly man, so ignored him.

3. Complications in relationships

(a) Being *taken advantage of.* My experience – somebody tricked me out of some money.

(b) *Hard to trust* people. If I don't know someone really well, I can't accept their help.

(c) *Not grasping subtleties* of social know-how in a close relationship. If a friend offers to buy me a drink, should I let them pay or not?

A glance at this set of notes tells you that there are three main difficulties to mention, and each of these is split down into a number of individual points, which are themselves emphasised. For example, in Section 1(a) you know you will be illustrating the fact that autistic people often take phrases literally which can put them in embarrassing situations and that you will be using your own experience of an event which happened to you in your past, perhaps when a person commented with a phrase like 'if you win the lottery, I'll eat my hat!', forcing you to wonder if they really would do so. Just the words 'eat my hat' in your preparations have been enough to jog your memory of the whole event, enabling you to explain the whole story/situation without putting it all down. Similarly, in Section 2(a), you may be talking about occasions when you had little concept of the social norm and waved your legs and arms around and spoke in a robotic manner in the local supermarket, grabbing everyone's attention for the wrong reason. The word 'robotic' has jogged your memory cells this time. Each part of a section will probably take you a couple of minutes to complete, and you should have a clear idea in your mind of the overall plan by picking out these key words at each stage. Remember that no one is perfect, and the audience will not expect you to be. Just getting through the first few experiences is an achievement in itself, as it proves to you that you can do it. As you become more confident, however, you will wish to learn the tricks of the trade on improving presentations and first impressions while actually at the venue. Let us now examine some of these in detail.

9.2 Communication: at the venue

9.2a Setting the scene

Once you arrive at your destination there will be several points to consider which, if you are in doubt, should be discussed with the person or people who asked you to give your presentation. For example, will you be standing up or sitting down while delivering your presentation? Is the room a small one where all the audience will be able to hear or see you easily? Or is it a larger one where you will need a microphone or other equipment? If so, make sure you know how to use them beforehand – you want to ensure people understand what you are delivering clearly and simply, whether it is a talk or a visual presentation. When I did my first talk with a microphone I found I was too tall for it and kept bending down – I then had to ask the organisers to adjust it. Try to check these things before the start of the presentation to save embarrassing delays later on. It is a good idea to have a drink handy as well (once again, ask the organiser), even if it is only a glass of water. Especially with longer events, it is very easy for your throat to feel very dry after a while, and you may find yourself coughing or losing your voice if you are not prepared.

9.2b The golden rule of a talk

The golden rule of any talk or presentation to others is to be able to arrange and deliver your points to the audience in a way that they will understand and can relate to. I have always said that no matter how knowledgeable people are in a topic, if they are professors with three or four science degrees and cannot communicate their ideas in an effective manner then they are not good teachers. The art of doing this can be much harder than one first thinks, because different approaches are needed in different situations. You may be discussing serious topics, or ones with more humour and light-heartedness. A younger audience may require shorter presentations or more frequent changes of topic, as otherwise their attention can easily wander. A more mature audience may be able to listen for more lengthy periods, but might be more interested in specific details or complicated facts, or may ask you unexpected questions to which you may not have all the answers. Your presentation may very well be timed as well, which makes the 'content' amount important. In this confusing array of different situations, how can one get a foothold without being overwhelmed by the occasion or seize up with nerves?

9.2c Keep things simple

The important thing to begin with is to keep things simple. For your first attempts at speaking, why not practise with just one other person, perhaps a member of your family or a well-trusted friend? Choose someone who can encourage you and give you advice when things go wrong. And do not make your speech too long, perhaps five or ten minutes at most. Once you have successfully mastered this and are feeling more confident, you can then start to try larger audiences and a longer talk. I can always remember my first proper 'oral' exam in one of my English classes in high school, at the age of about 16. I had hardly spoken to any other youngsters before this because of my vulnerability to being bullied and lack of confidence socially, and I felt like jelly just before the assessment. But I had researched my topic well and knew exactly what I wanted to say. For the next ten minutes or so I had to stand up in front of a small class of pupils and a handful of teachers and, despite feeling very nervous, managed to describe in detail the incredibly large scale of things in the universe, starting with our own solar system and then moving on to the stars. By the time I had told them that a beam of light travelling at more than 186,000 miles a second would take 100 millennia to cross the galaxy we live in from one side to the other, the audience seemed almost spellbound and totally focused. My English teacher congratulated me at the end, and I felt rather pleased, especially as I was one of the most fluent speakers there. The considerable factual knowledge of the sciences that autistic people often possess can become very useful when we are trying to entertain an audience!

9.2d Be aware of reception from audience while giving your presentation

Remember to open your display with a greeting – it may sound obvious but it can be forgotten when one is trying to think about a hundred other things. You may want to start with something like 'Good morning, ladies and gentlemen, my name is [your name] and I'm very pleased to be asked here today to give a presentation on "What is autism?"'. Obviously most presenters will have to refer to their cues on many occasions throughout their presentation but you should try to look at your audience as much as possible. If the number of people listening to you is large, you may have to move your head slightly from left to right as you look across the room. Doing this a number of times will ensure that there are instances when you are looking at each group of listeners, otherwise you may give the impression of constantly staring at one corner of the room.

It is usually possible to pick up hints on how you might be getting on by being aware of your audience's behaviour. If they are sitting quietly and looking contented or deeply interested in what you are saying, the chances are you are doing OK. On the other hand, if they are getting restless, perhaps with a lot of coughing, movement or conversation amongst themselves, it could be an indication that you have been taking too long on one item and should try to move onto the next topic before people get bored.

9.2e Provide variety to freshen your display

By explaining or showing your audience a number of different facts or situations, you stand a better chance of getting most people interested somewhere along the line than if you just keep to the same thing all the time. Remember that what interests one person may not interest another so much and vice versa.

Most major presentations have at least the following three sections:

1. a clear statement of exactly what you wish to describe and how you plan to divide it up throughout the time allowed

2. descriptions of the main characteristics of your chosen subject, perhaps by means of individual experience or examples

3. drawing conclusions from your research and giving advice to others on how to use the information that you have just given.

If I were to give a general talk on autism, I would probably start by explaining, from my point of view, what it is like to have the condition, using a number of examples to illustrate my points. This would set an overall flavour for the rest of the talk and give my audience an idea on what to expect next. Then, I would perhaps explain in detail some of my own life experiences and how I learnt to overcome the difficulties I encountered. Finally, I would consider how I could use my knowledge of these occurrences to explain to the audience how other autistic people could learn to cope with similar things happening to them, and what they and their carers or families can do in a practical sense to help spread knowledge and awareness of autism's characteristics and how to live with it. The saying 'variety is the spice of life' is very apt in the context of giving a good and interesting presentation. All of this can be delivered using pictures, drawings, photographs and equipment such as computers or electronic aids.

9.2f Learn through mistakes

As with many other things, we often learn more through our mistakes than when things are going well. It is important to realise that you will go wrong from time to time, and that things do not always go exactly to plan. It may seem embarrassing at the time, but the important thing is not to dwell on it too much but to move on as soon as you have dealt with the complication. Supposing you had accidentally knocked your glass of water over and had to stop for a moment to wipe the dampness away from your notes. You may just say, 'Sorry about that, audience – let's carry on'. However, another good way of 'covering up' a mistake, so to speak, can be to make a joke of it and laugh it off. It is often a good idea to throw in a bit of humour from time to time anyway in a talk, and a comment like 'There goes my drink – it shows I'm not awake yet!' may generate a relaxed atmosphere with a touch of light-heartedness which gives your listeners the message that you are not going to dwell on this incident for too long or let it disrupt the rest of your talk. Handling this minor misfortune in the correct way can make it far more likely to be forgotten quickly. You will also no doubt learn something yourself and remember, in your next presentation, to put your drink down on a separate table, say, where you will not be likely to knock it over.

9.2g Coping with nerves

Being a bit nervous before giving any kind of performance is perfectly normal, and indeed may very well improve your performance, as you will be keyed up and ready to concentrate fully on what you are doing. Excessive anxiety, however, can inhibit results. One way of reducing this anxiety is by having a thorough understanding of your chosen topic and being very familiar with it, so that in the back of your mind you will not run out of things to say or do and stand there like a zombie. I once delivered a talk on autism for about an hour, doing marvellously, and then shortly after that I won a sports award for tennis endeavour and was asked to give a brief two- or three-minute speech at the presentation awards. I almost literally 'froze', with no words coming out of my mouth simply because I had not prepared anything and was not familiar with what I was going to say.

Another problem could arise if you stutter, or have difficulty saying certain words. I used to have difficulty saying many words in English that started with the letter R and would call out a word like 'R-R-R-Remember'. The trouble is, the more you think about the fact that you have stuttered and the more the delay in the fluency of your speech goes on, the more conscious you are going to get and the more the audience is going to notice. To get out of this trap you could either say the word slowly, saying the 'R' first, or substitute another word with a similar meaning (in this case just say 'memorise' and people will probably know what you mean). If you are doing a presentation and find it difficult to speak or don't speak and use electronic equipment, facial expressions and gestures can really help.

9.2h Dealing with youngsters

The age range of your audience can be important, because it can determine the length and detail of your presentation, as well as the language used. Remember that complicated phrases such as 'social repertoire' which would be largely understood by an adult audience will probably not mean anything to younger children who have almost certainly never heard the term. Why not replace it by 'social sayings' or 'social know-how'? Another trap to avoid is to make reference to something that you recall as a youngster but that was probably no longer around by the time your audience reached the same age as you were then. I once used the film *Rainman* as an example of something that depicted the character-istics of autism, but most of my audience had never heard of it because the film was released before their time. I had to change my example to the character Martin in *Grange Hill*, a then-current show that my audience could relate to.

Although I have been concentrating mainly on autistic talks, there is no reason why we cannot talk or present about other subjects as well, providing we properly understand the material ourselves. Teaching and explaining mathematics has been an absorbing hobby for me over a number of years.

9.3 Communication: answering questions

It is often customary at some point in a presentation, especially towards the end, to have a question and answer session, where the audience can fire questions at you about the topics you have been discussing. This part can often seem more daunting to the autistic speaker than the rest of the event, because at least when you are delivering you are the one running the show and (you hope!) in control of what you are about to do, but questions coming from the audience could come in any form, and their unpredictable nature makes it hard to revise and prepare for. As a general rule, it is best to be honest if you really do not have any idea of an answer, although you may be able to make an educated guess or suggest alternative action which would enable them to find the information they require. Suppose for instance somebody asked you a difficult question involved with the medical aspects of autism. You might respond by saying, 'I don't have a detailed answer on me now, but you could contact the National Autistic Society who will advise you on how to obtain the necessary medical files/ material'. One more point – try to ensure that when a person is asking you a question that the rest of your audience has heard it, as in a big room many may not be able to. If necessary, repeat what the question was to everyone else before answering it. People with little communication through speech may need additional help in responding to questions.

Although you can never be totally sure what sort of questions will be asked, a thorough understanding of your chosen topic will give you confidence that you will be able to have a go at most of them. Another key point is not to spend too much time answering one question. Yes, perhaps go on for two or three minutes, but not much longer: you must give the others a chance too. On the other hand, you must try to be clear in your responses and answer the question asked, not the question that you might wish to answer. If somebody asked me, 'From your experience, what are the chief tell-tale signs to look for in recognising autism?' I would not proceed to spend the next half an hour explaining about how I used to pretend to be a robot, because however much it might have amused me I would be concentrating on only one factor. The person has asked for what *aspects* (as a plural) you can look for, so *brief* but *concise* mentioning of things such as lack of eye contact, spinning objects, lack of social interaction and taking everyday phrases literally would be required to give that person an *overall view* of what is required.

9.4 Writing

9.4a Getting started

Of course, not everyone will like the idea of presenting in front of large audiences. Some autistic people may not have a fluent or wide enough vocabulary or little speaking ability, or they might be rather shy and prefer to write down their thoughts on paper. Remember that almost anyone can pick up a newspaper or magazine to read, and this can be just as effective a way of spreading knowledge on autism to others as explaining it verbally. To get going, you might want to start by writing short stories for school magazines, articles for a local newsletter or paper, or perhaps a periodic magazine from your care manager's workplace (if you have one). Many people will be very interested to know about how your anxieties caused by your autism can affect your daily life.

Once you have produced the work in legible form, you then have to approach the team of people who organise the production of your article. Unless you are very confident, I would suggest checking this out with your teacher, your support worker or a trusted friend or family member first. You may have to attend an interview, where they could ask you quite detailed questions, and you need to think very carefully and state precisely what you would like to be published. You do not, for example want all your personal details (such as your address) released, unless you are absolutely certain you understand what the implications of this could be. Otherwise you might get some unexpected phone calls or knocks on the door of your house from people you do not know, or know very little about, for example.

9.4b Longer articles and books

If you are considering writing a major piece of work involving tens or even hundreds of pages, it is very important to plan ahead and have a clear idea of the overall framework of your proposal. Never mind the finer details of every individual point. The first thing to do is to draw up an initial draft (a clear breakdown into a number of different sections of work, with an indication of what needs to be done or what you are aiming for in each section, perhaps in the form of a short list or a number of examples). For instance, suppose you were inspired enough to want to write your autobiography. You might decide to divide your book up into chapters according to your age, and then think of, say, five or six key events in that part of your life that you wish to write about. A hypothetical reader might produce a draft something like this:

My autobiography

Working title

Dedication of book to my cousin Ruth

Initial draft of contents

Introduction

Chapter 1

1.1   Give my name and age

1.2   Describe objectives of book and for whom it is intended

1.3   Explain layout of book. Give reader overall impression of what to expect

1.4   Write about the characteristics of autism and how it might affect individuals

Chapter 2: My first five years

2.1   Family details; home location

2.2   Memories of feeling isolated; not mixing with other children, as my brothers and sisters did

2.3   Ability to remember number plates on cars from early age and other numerical details

2.4 Recurring dream that frightened me

2.5 Taking statements literally

2.6 How changes in routine upset me

Chapter 3: Years 6–8

3.1 Primary school experiences and my unusual factual knowledge

3.2 The time I got kept in after school for shouting

3.3 The upsetting period when Cousin Ruth died of cancer

3.4 My obsession with watching spinning objects for hours and how it affected others

3.5 How and when my disability was first diagnosed

3.6 My fear of loud ringing sounds, and how they startled me, after a bad experience

[And so on]

Not only is it a lot easier for you to memorise facts that you once thought of, and know which parts of your book you have done, and still need to do, but it also enables other people to get a basic picture in their mind about the structure of your book. This can be especially useful if you approach a publisher to ask them if they are interested in producing your work. If you can get the overall design to their liking, it is then much easier to correct or alter small sections or a simple chapter or two later on. If you had just written the book with no such pre-plan, you would be liable to lack coherent structure or flow to your book, and may repeat yourself on topics that you had already mentioned once, but forgotten that fact, as there was no easy way to find it in the text. In addition, any proposed publisher may not like the design of your book, and it is very hard to rewrite an entire book!

9.4c Book contract

Even if you are successful in being offered a contract for a book, this procedure alone could make you face some challenging decisions. The idea of a time limit might make you feel under pressure, especially if a substantial part of your script is not yet written. It is not always easy to judge how long a book will take to complete, particularly as you may have many other commitments in everyday life. Most contracts also contain a long list of legal rules on how the process will operate, and what this will mean for you. Some of these rules are quite complicated and you should ask a trusted adult for advice and get someone else to look through it with you *before* you sign it, if you are at all unsure of anything in its contents. Let us not be too negative, however! Anyone with autism who is in a position of having a book publication opportunity come their way is already in the top few per cent of individual achievers and should feel proud of themselves. They also should have enough confidence in their ability to overcome these difficulties and to be able to estimate *approximately* how long the book will take to complete. For practical purposes it is better to have a contract than not to have one, otherwise you could spend ages on your work and then the publisher may not have any place for it. On the other hand it is better to ask for an extension than to rush your work. Many publishers will offer extensions to any deadlines, provided you give them reasonable notice. This can significantly calm the nerves or fear of not finishing on time. So ask them! Be honest with your publisher. Explain your fears to them. You should be able to work out a plan together on how to proceed and minimise stress. Agree on a compromise, and then get on with it. You have a responsibility to inspire others with this great opportunity. You cannot afford to ignore that challenge, for the sake of all of us understanding autism better!

9.5 Using other methods to communicate

Finally, a brief mention of the fact that even if you are not able to stand up in front of others to give a talk or unable to write, this does not necessarily mean the end of all your hopes, as there are other ways of communicating with audiences and the like, not all of which are immediately obvious to the individual. If you can type on the keyboard of a computer then it should be possible to translate your thoughts electronically across a network, or perhaps over the Internet to groups of people with suitable devices to receive the messages. Although procedures like this are less common or well known than the more usual oral or written ways, you should never let any disability get in the way of being able to tell others your views in a presentation set-up. Once again you should seek advice from your family, friends or support personnel on the practicalities of performing a talk or demonstration with your individual circumstances. Some people have been very successful in producing publications with pictures, drawing, poems and video stories.

9.6 Media coverage: appearing on television and radio

Sometimes there may be opportunities to appear on TV or radio. This may also give opportunities to individuals to become more well known. If this happens, you may very well be asked to attend more prestigious events, and perhaps experience the thrill of appearing in the media. You could then ask for a copy of your programme, and keep it for ever as a memento of your great achievement. I appeared on the *QED* documentary programme on BBC1 back in 1995. The programme featured several aspects of my life then, including my university details, how I travelled about and my phobia about washing-machines flooding. This involved several meetings with the film crew, and it can be the ultimate test of nerves to feel you are talking fluently and looking good, knowing that thousands or even millions of people could be watching or listening to you. But remember, unless the programme is 'live', there will always be the chance to go back and film you again if you make a mistake or they are not satisfied with your response. If you do get the chance and say yes, you will have to be prepared to give up several hours of your time over a few days. I had to fit mine in during my degree studies in maths. Be patient too, even if the film crew ask you to repeat a scene several times so you can appear in the best possible way. It is well worth the effort for a perhaps once-in-a-lifetime chance to improve your fame. It can also be great fun!

9.7 Talking at national and world levels

This demands a combination of the skills already mentioned, and more, but remember that if you do get invited to give a presentation for such prestigious events you will no doubt already be a confident person in your own right and will able to meet the challenge. Many conferences (such as the international one at Leeds in 1995 which I attended, the biggest of its kind ever held at the time by the National Autistic Society) have fixed timetables with only a certain amount of time allowed for each person. So it is an important skill to be aware of how long your presentation is taking, and to have back-up plans in your mind with the ability to add bits of information or delete them, according to whether you are running ahead or behind time, and to know which bits to add/delete. For a really professional touch, it helps to memorise practically all your notes and cues, so that you are able to look at the audience and to make decisions in the blink of an eye on what or what not to say at different moments and situations in your talk.

CHAPTER 10

Dealing with Uncertainty

This chapter is about making decisions. At times in our lives we all have to take responsibility for making them. Have you ever got the feeling of starting a chain reaction of events as a result of one single decision, one that could be highly inconvenient for anyone and might seem like a nightmare for someone with autism? Let me tell you a story. I am a fully grown autistic man. I have learnt to adapt to many things in everyday life. I use public transport, perform public talks on autism, and play and teach tennis. But my own house is sacred to me. It is my place of safety – the one location in which I feel I can back away from the stresses of a perplexing world, unwind and relax. Any invasion of that privacy by others entering my dwelling causes me stress. I have always found this the hardest thing to cope with. Even my support worker and own family are interrogated. 'Have you touched my clean bath towel? Have you altered the state of any electrical item like my heater? Have you touched any of my food and drink?' The list is endless, and built up over the years through a period of mistrust and being taken advantage of by others, as well as suffering three burglaries in a former home. I became fanatical about cleanliness and insisted upon washing everything up as soon as everyone had left, as well as checking every mains plug.

10.1 The complications of mistrust

At least with people I know well I know deep down they will not deliberately do me any harm. I can always check my concerns with them, and record it on a piece of paper for reference later. But with other people, such as plumbers, it is not so easy. You cannot ask them, 'Have you touched the cables behind my TV or video recorder, and are they still safe to use?' because this would appear odd and against what is expected. You have instead to deal with the horror of uncertainty. And at one point in the recent past I was going to have to deal *extreme* uncertainty.

It all started by a seemingly trivial decision made in a couple of minutes. It ended up being a couple of months of horror. This is what happened. One of my bath taps had developed a slight drip. Not much, but just enough for me to notice and hear the occasional dripping sound at night. Autistic people can be very acutely affected by sounds. They notice things like this. It can plague their minds and will not go away. For days I was in two minds about what to do about it. If I phoned the council to ask for it to be fixed, I would have to let a stranger into my house. I would have to cope with the anxiety of knowing he could be touching anything. I knew I would have to spend hours cleaning up the house afterwards. But at least the tap would then be fixed. On the other hand, if I did not ask, these stresses would not happen. But then what if the tap got worse? I could be up half the night worrying about there being a flood, being just as anxious. It seemed a no-win situation.

10.2 The example of the dripping tap

10.2a The cause of the problem

I eventually decided, after a discussion with my support worker, to contact the council and ask them to come and fix the tap. It was just a simple washer, that is all. It should not take more than 20 minutes at the most once they came. This was on Wednesday. The council would contact me when they knew a time for it to be done, I was told. Well, the first thing I was to learn about most plumbers is that the word 'predictable' does not exist to them! They only turn up when you have gone out. And when you stay in, you can wait all day with no one arriving at all. Sure enough, just two days later, on Friday morning, I went out. I had not heard anything from the council and was assuming they would not come until the following week. When I returned home later in the day, a note had been put through my door. They had turned up, totally unannounced. Somewhere in the countless regulations of my contract to the council, a rule had stated that the priority ranking of my repair request meant a two-day wait. And to them, the two days were up. Unfortunately, I was no psychic. Already unsettled by this, I had to call several friends and the council to arrange a proper appointment for the following week.

After a few more days of the dripping tap, a man from the council did turn up. Now at least, I thought, I can put this all behind me. But hold on, what was this I was being told? 'We cannot just replace the washer I'm afraid, mate. New regulations demand that with the type of bath you have, we remove both your taps and replace them with completely new ones.' Suddenly the task had already got three times longer, with half my bath tub unscrewed and taken to bits as the man struggled to put the new taps on. But the worst was yet to come. The chap had of course drained my hot water tank while he worked on the taps. Now for some reason the tank was not filling up again. Something was wrong, terribly wrong! After what seemed like hours, with the plumber in desperation at being unsuccessful at finding the cause of the problem, he called another plumber in to seek advice. What had happened was that my entire hot water tank had got gunged up with material that was preventing it from working properly. 'I'm afraid,' said the second plumber, 'that we shall have to get you a completely new hot water tank! And we can't do that for a couple of days, at least'. It was now after 5 p.m. The whole day had gone. Soon after, both plumbers left, leaving me without any hot water! Far from being resolved, this situation was getting almost unbearable for me. It was going to be a long 48 hours.

10.2b The dilemma intensifies

As soon as the men had gone I desperately tried to clean every tap and work surface in the house. That is extra difficult if you do not have any hot water. They say that necessity is the mother of invention. It rang true here. I had to put myself on a higher level of coping. Sometimes one is forced to face those fears. The autistic person who copes well with independence is one who can learn through these experiences how to deal with them and emerge a stronger individual for next time around. Somehow I got through those two days. Then one of the council men returned. Surely now, I thought, they would put the new tank in and this would all be over? Not on your life! 'Really sorry,' I was told, 'We've looked everywhere for your required tank design, and can't find it. We'll have to order from further afield'. I felt numb. Because of their commitments and mine, nothing was now going to be possible until the following week. A whole week without hot water! My normal schedule simply fell to pieces for that week. This was the middle of winter, the time when you most need hot water. I had never used a kettle to boil water for fear of electrical equipment and burning myself (a fear I have had all my life), and I did not feel able to start now. How on earth was I going to manage to bath, keep clean and wash things up?

On two or three occasions a couple of good friends of mine let me go to their homes in the evening so that I could have a proper bath. Even here I had some concerns. I insisted on taking my own soap for fear of it not being hygienic for them if I used theirs. I carried my own towel up there for the same reason. But the hot bath was paradise. You will never appreciate it so much as when you have been deprived of it for a while. There were also other times in that week when I felt too tired or my friends were busy and I could not make it over to their place. Rather than go without, I forced myself to have a bath once a day in cold water. I even washed my hair a couple of times with a jug of freezing water! I would far rather do that than face the fear of the electric kettle. Our phobias with autism can run very deep. At least it can make us be decisive. This for me was the lesser of two evils. The way I felt I would be most able to cope. Then, after what seemed like for ever, the following Monday arrived. I had been scheduled for the first call from the council that day. They had now finally found the new tank. I stared at it. It looked enormous. Much bigger than the other one, I thought, as soon as they arrived. The old tank was quickly removed. Directly after this had been done, one of the council men was staring at my cupboard with a very worried look on his face. What on earth now, I thought?

10.2c To the depths of despair!

My original hot water tank had been set in a small cupboard in my kitchen. A cupboard with a narrow doorway, that was only just big enough to squeeze that tank through. The new tank design was much bigger. And it would not go in! 'Not again. Not another week without hot water!' flashed through my worry thoughts. 'Well,' said the plumber, 'there's only one thing for it'. And he got to work. For the whole day. Not putting the new tank in. That was not until evening time. The rest of the time was spent demolishing half of my kitchen wall to create a gap large enough to do so! While he hammered away for hour after hour I spent most of the time lying on my lounge floor, reduced to tears, not knowing when this was going to end, if ever. I tended to go out for dinner in order to avoid confronting my electrical phobia as manifest in cookers and kettles, and also as the only way to meet friends and see other people for emotional support and break the otherwise terrible loneliness of staying at home all day. Now I was being deprived even of that as I'd had to stay in far too long with the plumber, and all the places I usually went to were already shut. At 8.30 that evening, after he finally left, the job still was not complete, and I had only partial hot water. That was despite the plumber doing me a favour by working later than he really had to. He would have to come back the following morning to carry on. I was already in panic mode. Once someone autistic gets like this, they can imagine almost anything. 'What if something went wrong tomorrow as well? And then the next day? What if I was stuck in a whole week or even longer while they completed the work? Would my life ever be the same again?', I lamented to myself.

Tuesday morning finally came. I had prepared for the worst. I had cancelled all other commitments for that week. I had arranged for friends to come round to my house to give me food to live on. And yet the plumber seemed to make good progress. By lunchtime he appeared to have finished. Except, I was told that 'you have to expect a few problems and complications with a brand new tank'. I did not actually quite believe he had gone. Then I went into the kitchen. This room had always been the one I was most anxious to keep clean, having all the food and drink in it. Now a thick layer of dust lay over everything. Bits of wood were scattered all over the floor. And my sacred washing-up bowl, the one item above all else to keep spotless…had been placed under the dirty tank to catch any water! I spent the rest of the day cleaning everything up. At least nearly everything. Those items I did not clean then I got help with cleaning the following day from my support worker. Then a couple of days of relative calm. But even then I was on edge. The new tank made some different sounds while it was settling in. But at least it worked properly. Or did it? The nightmare was not yet done.

10.2d The agony continues

Just a few weeks later, having remained unsettled about the loud hissing of the new tank, I was awoken by a terrible bubbling sound in the kitchen. As I opened the door I thought there was a fire. There was steam and dripping water all over the window, and water was leaking out from the bottom of the hot water tank. The tank had been overheating and I had to call out the emergency plumber who could not do anything much except isolate the supply. This was Sunday, of course. That is the other rule you will find. Things usually only go wrong at the weekend or bank holidays when plumbers are hard to find! Once again, an anxious wait until Monday lay ahead of me, not knowing what to expect. Another sleepless night. Monday morning arrived, so did the plumber. Another plumber? Well, actually, an electrician to be precise! This time a faulty thermostat was to blame. It did not take too long to fix. After I had spent the rest of Monday cleaning up the house (yet again!), on Tuesday afternoon I finally started to relax a tiny bit. *At last* I thought. A whole day without having to think about plumbers. Let's go for a nice hot bath, and wash my worries away. I turned on the hot tap. Only a little trickle of water for a few moments, and then…nothing! Not a single drop of hot water could be seen even with the tap full on. Off we go again! Emergency plumber number two was called round late on Tuesday night. He looked and looked. What could it be? A blocked water pipe? An air bubble? Then he realised what had happened. The previous visitor had forgotten to turn the valve back on. The tank had been unable to refill itself as a result! That was all. We had been looking for ages for other problems that were not there.

It took me another week to recover fully and get back to even half a normal routine. My support worker and I had to see the funny side of it. One simple choice to have one tiny tap washer on one small tap in the bathroom about two months ago had produced a chain reaction of events, the unpredictability of which had tested my ability to cope and function well to the limit. I had already been through an earlier incident when there was a loose tile on my roof that let water leak into the larder. That had also taken weeks to resolve. I had sat for hours staring at the bucket on the larder floor put there to catch the water (well some of it anyway!). Every night I had to mop up the wet that missed the bucket. And of course this happened during a period of really heavy continuous rain. I decided, after these two incidents, to get together with my support worker and discuss contingency plans I could follow in case this sort of thing happens again. I have been talking a lot about myself so far in this chapter. But this is a book designed to help other autistic people. So let's consider a few points about plumbers that I learnt through my experiences, and that others in my position may find useful.

10.3 Is a plumber really required?

Whenever you discover a problem in your home, your first priority is to decide how urgent the situation is and whether it definitely needs a plumber, electrician or other repair man to fix it. Many small things like a really squeaky door or loose shelf may be repaired by you (at worst with a friend or social worker) with a few drops of oil or simple DIY. On the other hand, a leaking hot water tank demands immediate attention. If you live in a council dwelling, major incidents requiring plumbers and the like will normally be done through them: you contact the council first and they then contact a plumber. Otherwise it will depend on circumstances such as the nature and severity of the problem and on legal technicalities. Your tenancy agreement and/or landlord should be able to tell you who is responsible for rectifying the problem. If you are at all unsure about how to deal with an occurrence, you should contact the people responsible for your welfare (this could be your family, a social worker or social service office, or the council directly, if applicable). Do contact someone though, otherwise the situation could get much worse.

10.4 Be ready for unpredictability

One very common criterion for autistic people is their wish to have an ordered and definite structure to their day, and to know exactly when things are going to happen. All this is likely to go out of the window as far as plumbers are concerned. It is virtually impossible to get a precise time, and even the prediction of a 'morning' or 'afternoon' call is not always followed. If you have been asked to wait in through the morning and duly do so, they will probably turn up one minute before lunch. *But* if you pop out for two minutes to buy a paper, the chances are they will come as soon as you have gone! So one needs to be firm and decisive both with the repair people and with yourself about how to proceed. If you have waited in half the morning for a morning call with no one showing up, why not call the council again and ask them to confirm that the plumber definitely is coming? Or decide to wait in until 2 p.m. in case they got held up with a previous job – this can often happen, especially if they are asked to undertake a task like replacing a hot water tank (we know all about that now, don't we?). One way of avoiding this sort of hold-up is to ask for the 'first call of the day', although you will have to be prepared to be up quite early (before 8 a.m. on occasions) and the appointment could still be affected by heavy traffic. If you have to go out later, phone the council again to tell them this and discuss another appointment. Remember that very few plumbers would turn up for work after 5 p.m. for non-emergency repairs.

10.5 Be ready – have your house prepared

While there may be little that an autistic individual can do to elim-inate all anxiety while a repair job is taking place, there are plenty of things that can be done before the repair man arrives. It is often a good idea to take items you do not wish them to handle away from the areas that they are likely to be working in. So if you do not want cartons of paint or pieces of wood stacked in your spotless washing-up bowl, why not move the bowl into another room out of sight of the plumbers? Similarly, if you use some glasses or mugs for drinking, why not wash them up and put them away instead of leaving them lying around to be knocked over or splashed with paint? Mind you, bear in mind that plumbers like to drink too, especially with long tiring repairs that take most of the day, and if you are able to offer them a drink and some biscuits then do so, but this is not a legal requirement, just a friendly gesture if you are up to it. There is no harm in helping out a bit in things like telling them where the stopcock is in your house or turning a tap on for them, but you should never have to do anything that you feel really uncomfortable with. Ultimately it is their responsibility to finish the repair. If, in addition you often rely on eating out under normal circumstances, you should either make sure you have enough provisions in your house the day before or make prior arrangements with friends to bring some food or drink round to you, rather than waiting and then going hungry all day because you have none of your favourite cookies left and cannot go out to buy them. Try to avoid leaving valuables lying around such as jewellery or money – put them out of sight.

10.6 Make waiting time productive

No matter how frustrating it may be to be stuck inside waiting for plumbers, or even after they have arrived and are getting on with their work – especially if the sun is shining outside, pleading with you to go out – it will not do you any good to sit and fret about the situation. On the contrary, it is probably the worst thing you can do, because the more your mind is free to wander about how much you are wishing to be outside with your friends, the more depressing things can seem. So keep your mind occupied. There are plenty of things that can be done while indoors. Why not write that letter to your long-lost friend in the United States, as you have promised you would weeks ago and never yet got round to it? Or watch that video you had for your birthday and never got round to seeing? If you are studying a course at college or university, this could be an opportunity to do some revision. Doing something productive with this waiting time will not only take your mind off the frustrations of the plumbers, but will also give you a sense that the day has not gone to waste and that you have something to show for it. You should also realise that once this job is fixed, with any luck it will not trouble you any more, and that you will become a more experienced and confident person in having dealt with it successfully.

10.7 Check things are OK at the end of the repairs

If you have any major queries such as 'Is my water working normally?' or 'Is my heating now safe to use?' after it has been checked out, you can always ask the plumber as they leave, to put your mind at rest. Do not keep them half an hour, though, with an encyclopaedia of questions – remember that plumbers have homes to go to as well, and they will want to get to them, particularly when they are exhausted after a long day. Quite often they will tell you the important things or instructions that you need to know or follow anyway, before they leave. After they have left, it is a good idea to clean up the work area where they have been during the day, even if it is a simple wipe down with a damp cloth or a quick vacuum. Remember that dust can settle on surfaces, especially after tools like electrical drills have been used. Be particularly careful about stray nails or screws or other sharp objects that may have been left undetected on tables, chairs or on the floor. They can be responsible for a nasty cut otherwise. Keep an eye on electrical switches too, and do not be surprised if you find an extra light left on or a tap not turned off properly. Other people may not be as particular as you are in wanting things exactly as they normally are. If the repairs are done through the council you will not usually have to pay for the work, although there are a few exceptions, and with private plumbers the situation could be very different. Always check with a trusted adult *before* a plumber visits you if you are at all unsure about their trustworthiness or whether you owe money and how much. Never let yourself be cheated out of cash.

CHAPTER 11

Autism in a Nutshell

The time has now come to summarise what the reader can learn through the experiences I have described throughout this book, so that we individuals with autistic spectrum disorders (ASD) can use and apply our new-found knowledge to live more fulfilling lives. There are a number of key factors that surface again and again, involving our behavioural patterns and anxieties, which tend to cause difficulty or misunderstanding from others. These include:

- *Levels of anxiety* – As was pointed out in Chapter 2, the intensely high levels of anxiety of those of us with ASD over what seem to others to be trivial things is often completely unappreciated. Moreover, we usually find that different individuals will worry about different things, and what works for calming down one of us may not work for another. It is not just the physical aspects of coping with life's challenges that need to be considered, but also the verbal and emotional interpretation of social interaction. It can be very disheartening for care workers and the like, who may initially feel they have mastered some of one client's characteristics, only to find that many of these apparent rules go out of the window when they start working with another client. One ASD individual may, under certain circumstances, even appear to function in two different ways, a normal coping mode and a worried panic state when things are not going well.

- *Mistrust of people* – In my own experience there have been many occasions when a fear of the unknown or of being taken advantage of has prevented me from attending or making progress with social events. Even among good friends, a fairly minor argument or disagreement can be very frightening for us ASD individuals, as we may start to doubt our own ability to socialise adequately or feel concerned about the continuing loyalty of our friend if that friend is annoyed, fearing that perhaps the friend may want to get back at us somehow or do us some harm. Many of us with ASD can find it extremely difficult to judge how serious or trivial such a falling-out might be. We may completely overreact and start mistrusting someone dear to us who would never do us any harm or equally not pick up hints when something is more serious and how upset a friend could be.

- *When your helpers fear the unknown* – As well as having difficulties yourself socially as someone with ASD, both with your friends and care staff, do not be surprised if you encounter prejudice from others. The bottom line is that many outsiders can fear what they do not understand and will tend to shy away from it whenever possible, not necessarily because they deliberately do not want to help, but rather because they are concerned that they cannot give aid in the right way. This situation could occur in the cases of family members, social workers and organisations with other people in authority as well as friends, although at least you could say in these cases that these people care about how they care for you! This is far better than having them barging in to assist in a way that they feel appropriate, without any regard to whether their method of assistance is even remotely close to a sound and correct form of help.

11.1 Stepping forward

There is much that can be done in a practical sense, by those in authority, to make the world easier for us. Already, much progress has been made – just 30 years ago, the term 'autism' was hardly known, and as a youngster, I attended what was then about the only help unit in the country specifically built for ASD individuals. Currently, many more specific help units have been set up in a number of counties, both for those at school age and more recently for those attending some universities and higher educational establishments, as well as adult day centres and care homes. We have finally begun to start spreading awareness and reducing the stigma associated with our condition, and proved that it does not mean a life deprived of social or academic opportunities. However, there is plenty of scope for improvement.

11.2 How others can make our lives easier

11.2a Different organisations should work in unison

In my view, the most important point to make on how to make further progress is that different sources of input from society, such as health and social services, parents, university personnel and local authorities, should attempt to work with each other to assist us in living with ASD. Too often progress may be made in one or two of these sources by a number of us but then, owing to a lack of communication or misuse of available resources, such achievements may not be given due praise or notice, and consequently opportunities for further developments can be reduced. Instead we should have an easily accessible specialised team of ASD professionals in every local authority. Such a team should preferably have a single referral point and be instantly recognisable, as parents are often concerned or baffled as to where to turn to for help, and other help sources will find it easier to get involved in working together. In order to allow for this, training programmes should be made readily available in each local area, catering for both parents and professionals.

11.2b *The necessity of a coherent structure*

The training for our teachers will need to be very intense and continuous, to allow these 'student' teachers to experience first-hand
working with several differently affected ASD people, which will
ensure that they have really got to grips with the main forms of
behavioural patterns under varying circumstances. Each local
team of ASD professionals should consist of staff from businesses
such as health services, educational establishments and social
facilities coordination, all working together to ensure that suitable
care plans are set up for each one of us with the condition. In
addition, a separate worker should be appointed to each family
concerned. It will be this one worker who will play a key role in
checking the suitability of such a care plan and will be able to
make contact with the area coordinator for ASD to that effect. Of
course, putting all these things in place can take time and money,
but all that is needed are the will and a sensible, correct use of the
necessarily limited available resources.

11.2c *Flexibility in the method of aid*

Early identification of the presence of ASD is important and I
mentioned this Chapter 2; it is also good for authorities to be
flexible in their training programmes and allow for the fact that
each of us with ASD will develop personal strategies for coping
with the challenges that life can throw out. More information on
sources of aid can be found in the listing at the end of the book
(Appendix 2). Sporting activities and games that involve
teamwork can be especially challenging, since by their very definition a certain amount of social understanding from others is
required (see Chapter 8). This is where a one-to-one support
system can prove invaluable to enable us with ASD to become
involved and 'fit in' with the activity, while continuing our
learning process through practice. I believe if you show good
behaviour and results you should always receive plenty of praise.
A tempting treat such as your favourite chocolate for the best per-

former of a given activity or exercise offered by your teacher can often be a great incentive to keep you fully concentrated! I can recall several similar occurrences during the time I was involved in coaching sport.

11.2d Help in education

We have seen how important it is for others to be aware of ASD at all centres of education (Chapter 7) and for the appropriate facilities to be available, but in addition let us not forget that we shall also need the necessary staff member to be trained, and such training should be available nearby. No amount of physical resources will be much good for a group of untrained teachers or ones with no experience of our condition. For a person like us, opportunities for socialising can often be just as crucial as academic support, and I hope that more social activities and clubs will become more ASD-friendly, with awareness of the condition growing nationally. Also, remember that, especially in educational establishments, there needs to be access to trained personnel concentrating on the specific individual requirements of people with ASD, such as occupational therapists, psychologists, and language and communication experts.

11.3 A lasting message from this book

The important thing to note about the events I describe in this book is to *be and think positive!* We have seen how a number of dramas can unfold in everyday life for an ASD individual, such as the plumbing experiences I went through in Chapter 10, but always at the end of the day we illustrate how one can learn to live through the experience and become a stronger and more experienced individual, being more able to cope mentally with similar occurrences in the future. This is the lasting message that I wish to make. There is no reason why ASD people cannot master and learn to live through what they find challenging; no matter how hard things may seem at the time, it is important to realise that in the process of getting through them, you will be able to find a feeling of true fulfilment and confidence with your life, in becoming more independent and with the knowledge that you will no doubt inspire others in their position to do likewise.

11.4 A final thought

A certain amount of common sense has to be used while attempting to work towards and achieve the goals mentioned above. There is no way that we can expect everything to happen at once, and many of the requirements, such as the training processes, will involve a great deal of hard work and organisation from our adult helpers. The rewards duly come, however, when we start reaping dividends from our efforts, transforming step by step our ASD lifestyles from an existence full of mental health problems to a successful integration into society. If even one such life can be altered for the better it has got to be worth all the effort (just imagine if it were you!). More likely, hundreds or even thousands of us could be transformed for the better simply through enough investment and careful use of resources. If all the major countries were able to embark upon similar programmes of support and awareness, we could easily see an increased level of awareness on a global scale with those people helped being numbered in the millions. As a person with ASD myself who has made the transformation, I find that there is no greater incentive to work towards helping others with ASD than watching the sheer joy on their faces when they find out what it is like to be happy, confident, independent and able to pursue their interests without prejudice. We should all try to share some of the responsibility of ensuring that our friends with autistic spectrum disorder live as fulfilling a life as is practically possible.

Fun with Numbers!

This appendix involves the study of mathematics and will be of interest both to other autistic individuals with a love of maths, and also any parents, carers and social workers with a decent background (roughly A-level) in the subject. It is clearly optional and can be omitted by those not interested, as it is largely independent of the text in the rest of this book. The main goal of the work is to illustrate how apparently simple properties and problems in maths can become progressively more and more complex as a result of noticing small details, these often going unnoticed by the average person but being picked up by an autistic mind which will often focus in on one particular point. To justify the chapter's inclusion in a book on autism, let us point out that this act of 'making a mountain out of a molehill' is not restricted to a study of the scenarios here, but can occur in virtually any everyday occurrence or task that an autistic person might face, e.g. dressing up for an interview – for example, 'Do I put the shirt on first, or the tie? Do I tuck the collar in or put the jacket on first? What order should I do the buttons up – top to bottom, or bottom to top?' Thus the chapter serves to illustrate the fact that while considering every possible outcome can make autistic people brilliant scientists or mathematicians, the same rigid way of thinking can make everyday practical tasks normally taken for granted by others a nightmare of complexity.

Let us initially restrict our domain to the positive real numbers, and with this in mind, let us define a function:

$$f: R^+ \rightarrow R^+; f(x) = x^x$$

where x can take any value we choose within this domain. Recall that a number a raised to the power of a positive integer b is the product of b such numbers, and denoting the result by c we can write

$$c = a \times a \times a \times ... \times a$$

there being b number a's multiplied together. The number a is known as the bth root of c, since it requires the product of b such numbers a to obtain c. Finally a number d raised to the power of a rational fraction k/l is defined as the lth root of d raised to the power of k. So for example, let $a = 2$, and $b = 3$, then $c = 2 \times 2 \times 2$ (known as 2 cubed or $2^3 = 8$) and if $a = 3$ and $b = 4$, then $c = 3^4 = 3 \times 3 \times 3 \times 3 = 81$. Also if $k = 2$ and $l = 3$ with $d = 8$ then $8^{2/3} = (2)^2$, since 2 is the cube root of 8, and $(2)^2 = 2 \times 2 = 4$. Returning to our function f let us work out some values of the function with different inputs.

$$f(2) = 2^2 \text{ which by definition is } 2 \times 2 = 4 \text{ (with } a = b = 2)$$

$$f(3) = 3^3 \text{ which by definition is } 3 \times 3 \times 3 = 27 \text{ (with } a = b = 3)$$

$$f(4) = 4^4 = 4 \times 4 \times 4 \times 4 = 256 \text{ (with } a = b = 4) \text{ and so on.}$$

Notice how the value of the function increases very rapidly as we increase the input. Consider the case where $x = 10$.

$$f(10) = 10^{10} = 10 \times 10 \times 10 \times 10 \times 10 \times 10 \times 10 \times 10 \times 10 \times 10$$

$$= 10{,}000{,}000{,}000$$

Let's see what happens if we use a fraction as input.

$$f\left(\tfrac{1}{2}\right) = \left(\tfrac{1}{2}\right)^{\frac{1}{2}} = \sqrt{\left(\tfrac{1}{2}\right)}$$

This can be written in equivalent form as $\frac{\sqrt{2}}{2}$ which is approximately equal to 0.7071

Also $f\left(\tfrac{3}{4}\right) = \left(\tfrac{3}{4}\right)^{\frac{3}{4}} = \left[\sqrt[4]{\left(\tfrac{3}{4}\right)}\right]^3$

which is approximately 0.8059 ($d = \tfrac{3}{4}$, $k = 3$, $l = 4$) and

$$f\left(\tfrac{15}{16}\right) = \left(\tfrac{15}{16}\right)^{\tfrac{15}{16}} = \left[\sqrt[16]{\tfrac{15}{16}}\right]^{15} \approx 0.9413 \ (d = \tfrac{15}{16}, k = 15, l = 16)$$

An inspection of this function by calculus reveals that its minimum value occurs when $x = \tfrac{1}{e}$, and this minimum value is approximately 0.6922 (note e is a special mathematical constant approximately equal to 2.7183).

As we increase our input value from $\tfrac{1}{e}$ so the magnitude of our output will also increase. What is perhaps less known is that as we decrease our input value below $\tfrac{1}{e}$ (but still greater than zero) the function actually increases the smaller the input amount we select, these functional values tending to 1 (and not zero as many people might think) although 0^0 will always remain undefined.

$$f\left(\tfrac{1}{100}\right) \approx 0.9550, f\left(\tfrac{1}{10000}\right) \approx 0.9991, \text{ and } f\left(\tfrac{1}{100000}\right) \approx 0.9999$$

Now we are going to inspect one of those tiny but crucial details mentioned at the start of this chapter that often go unnoticed by the unwary. You may have noticed that the result of multiplying a set of real numbers together is always the same whatever the order in which we carry out this task. For example, $(3 \times 4) \times 5 = 3 \times (4 \times 5)$ irrespective of whether we evaluate 3×4 first and then multiply by 5, or evaluate 4×5 first and then multiply by 3. Moreover, we can interchange the numbers, e.g. $3 \times 4 \times 5 = 4 \times 5 \times 3 = 5 \times 3 \times 4$. That these facts are not true for all mathematical structures may not be immediately obvious. Consider the expression

$$x^{x^x}$$

This expression as it stands might be argued to be ambiguous, and not define a function. For does it mean evaluate x^x first and then raise x to the power of this result, or does it mean raise the result to the power of x? Let us define two functions that do make sense, as the order of preference is made clear by bracketing terms. Let

$$g: R^+ \rightarrow R^+; g(x) = \left(x^x\right)^x \text{ and } h: R^+ \rightarrow R^+; h(x) = x^{\left(x^x\right)}$$

At first sight it may appear that $g = h$ for all x. After all

$$g(1) = (1^1)^1 = 1^1 = 1 \quad h(1) = 1^{\left(1^1\right)} = 1^1 = 1 \quad \text{thus } g(1) = h(1) \text{ and}$$

$$g(2) = \left(2^2\right)^2 = 4^2 = 16 \quad h(2) = 2^{\left(2^2\right)} = 2^4 = 16 \quad \text{so } g(2) = h(2)$$

Looks can be deceptive however, and these input choices are the exception rather than the rule. Normally, $g(x) \neq h(x)$, indeed for large x, function h increases far more rapidly than function g. For instance

$$g(3) = \left(3^3\right)^3 = 27^3 = 19683 \text{ but } h(3) = 3^{\left(3^3\right)} = 3^{27}$$

which is approximately equal to 7625597485000, a vastly greater number.

$$g(4) = \left(4^4\right)^4 = 256^4 = 4294967296 \quad \text{but} \quad h(4) = 4^{\left(4^4\right)} = 4^{256}$$

which is approximately

1340780792000000000000000000000000000000000000000000
0000000000000000000000000000000000000000000000000000
0000000000000000000000000000000000000000000000000000
00000

that is $1.340780792 \times 10^{154}$

So beware of functions that look identical to one another but are not!

The normal convention with an expression such as x^{x^x} is to start from the top layer and work downwards. So for example

$$x^{x^x} = x^{\left(x^x\right)}; \quad x^{x^{x^x}} = x^{\left(x^{\left(x^x\right)}\right)}; \qquad x^{x^{x^{x^x}}} = x^{\left(x^{\left(x^{\left(x^x\right)}\right)}\right)}$$

However, we can easily define other functions from the same expressions by simply changing the order of our brackets and evaluations. Considering the 4-layer powered expression

$$x^{x^{x^x}}$$

we see that there are four possibilities – let us denote them as follows

$$L_1 : R^+ \rightarrow R^+; \qquad L_1(x) = \left(\left(x^x\right)^x\right)^x$$

$$L_2 : R^+ \to R^+; \qquad\qquad L_2(x) = \left(x^{\left(x^x \right)} \right)^x$$

$$L_3 : R^+ \to R^+; \qquad\qquad L_3(x) = x^{\left(\left(x^x \right)^x \right)}$$

$$L_4 : R^+ \to R^+; \qquad\qquad L_4(x) = x^{\left(x^{\left(x^{\left(x^x \right)} \right)} \right)}$$

Evaluating each function in the case when $x = \frac{3}{2}$ we obtain the following results correct to 4 decimal places

$$L_1(1.5) = 3.9292 \quad L_2(1.5) = 3.0567 \quad L_3(1.5) = 2.7446$$

$$L_4(1.5) = 2.3490$$

a different result each time. A similar expression in x with five levels of powers will generate nine distinct functions as we evaluate brackets in different orders, three of them being

$$M_1 : R^+ \to R^+; \qquad\qquad M_1(x) = \left(\left(\left(x^x \right)^x \right)^x \right)^x$$

$$M_2 : R^+ \to R^+; \qquad\qquad M_2(x) = \left(x^{\left(x^x \right)} \right)^{\left(x^x \right)}$$

$$M_3 : R^+ \to R^+; \qquad\qquad M_3(x) = x^{\left(x^{\left(x^{\left(x^{\left(x^x \right)} \right)} \right)} \right)}$$

The fascinating fact is that as we increase the number of levels of powers the possibility of possible functions you can generate will increase also, so that it should be possible to produce thousands, or even millions of distinct functions from a simple power tower with n levels in variable x, provided n is large enough! Any mathematicians amongst you might find it a challenge to try and find a general formula for the number of such distinct functions from an 'n' level power tower in terms of n. To this day I have not yet met anyone who has managed it. Dare we make a comparison with the above expressions and learning all the rules of socialising – what starts off seemingly simple gets more and more complicated the longer you think about it!

It is time to broaden our domain of numbers to enable us to deal with our next discussion, locating roots of polynomial equations. If we restrict ourselves to the positive reals, the simple equation

$$3x + 2 = 0$$

has no solution, but if we allow for negative real numbers the solution $x = -\frac{2}{3}$ is soon found. Having made this one extension, let us now make another, and allow for complex numbers in our domain. Recall that the general form for a complex number is given by $z = a + bj$ where a and b are real numbers and $j^2 = -1$. It is usual to replace x by z when complex numbers are involved, but the solution of

$$3z + 2 = 0$$

is still $z = -\frac{2}{3}$, in this case $a = -\frac{2}{3}$ and $b = 0$ in our general form for z.

We will be considering the general polynomial of degree n

$$a_n z^n + a_{n-1} z^{n-1} + a_{n-2} z^{n-2} + \ldots \qquad + a_2 z^2 + a_1 z + a_0 = 0$$

where $a_i (0 \le i \le n)$ are constants, n is a positive integer and z is a complex number

this can be written more compactly as $\sum_{i=0}^{n} a_i z^i \ (a_n \neq 0)$

An important result in mathematics (known as the fundamental theorem of algebra) shows that an equation of the above form has, in general, exactly n roots (although some of these may be repeats). So an equation of the second degree (a quadratic) has two solutions, an equation of third degree (a cubic) has three solutions, an equation of fourth degree has four solutions, and so on. Let us look at some examples

Example 1   let $n = 2$, $a_0 = 12$; $a_1 = -7$, $a_2 = 1$. Our equation is

$$z^2 - 7z + 12 = 0$$

which can be factorised to

$$(z - 3)(z - 4) = 0$$

so in this case our equation has two real roots $z = 3$ and $z = 4$.

Example 2   let $n = 2$, $a_0 = 25$, $a_1 = -6$, $a_2 = 1$. We have

$$z^2 - 6z + 25 = 0$$

which can be written

$$[z - (3 + 4j)][z - (3 - 4j)] = 0$$

so in this case we have two complex roots $z = 3 + 4j$ and $z = 3 - 4j$.

It is often taught in maths classes that if a quadratic equation has any complex roots they always occur as a pair of complex conjugates, that is, in the forms $a + bj$ and $a - bj$, but what may be less well known (another one of those small details autistic people can notice!) is that this is only true if the constants a_0, a_1 and a_2 are all real.

Example 3   let $n = 2$, $a_0 = 10 - 2j$, $a_1 = -5$, $a_2 = 1$. We have

$$z^2 - 5z + (10 - 2j) = 0$$

Here also we have two complex solutions $z = 3 + 2j$ and $z = 2 - 2j$, but these are not complex conjugates of each other (a_0 is not a real constant here).

Example 4   let $n = 3$, $a_0 = -1$, $a_1 = a_2 = 0$, $a_3 = 27$. We thus have the cubic equation

$$27z^3 - 1 = 0$$

and we anticipate three roots. Since $27z^3 - 1 = (3z - 1)(9z^2 + 3z + 1)$ the equation can be written in the form

$$(3z - 1)(9z^2 + 3z + 1) = 0$$

so either $3z - 1 = 0 \Rightarrow z = \frac{1}{3}$ (this is perhaps the more obvious solution, and indeed with real numbers it is the only solution) or $9z^2 + 3z + 1 = 0$, which with our complex number system gives

$$z = -\frac{1}{6} + \frac{\sqrt{3}j}{6} \text{ or } z = -\frac{1}{6} - \frac{\sqrt{3}j}{6}$$

so the full solution set of the equation is $\frac{1}{3}, -\frac{1}{6}(1+\sqrt{3}j), -\frac{1}{6}(1-\sqrt{3}j)$

Note also that here the complex roots are conjugates of each other (all the coefficients of the equation are real).

Example 5   let $n = 4$, $a_0 = -1$, $a_1 = 2j$, $a_2 = 0$, $a_3 = 2j$, $a_4 = 1$. Our equation is

$$z^4 + 2jz^3 + 2jz - 1 = 0$$

This equation can be expressed in the form $g(z)(z-\alpha)^p = 0$ where in this case $g(z) = z-j$, $\alpha = -j$, and $p = 3$, and thus has a repeated root of multiplicity 3. The solution set of the equation being $\{-j, -j, -j, j\}$.

Example 6   let $n = 10$; $a_0 = -84$, $a_1 = -72$, $a_2 = -184$, $a_3 = -168$, $a_4 = -133$, $a_5 = -138$, $a_6 = -33$, $a_7 = -48$, $a_8 = 1$, $a_9 = -6$, $a_{10} = 1$. Our equation is

$z^{10} - 6z^9 + z^8 - 48z^7 - 33z^6 - 138z^5 - 133z^4 - 168z^3 - 184z^2 - 72z - 84 = 0$, which has solutions (after a rather tedious investigation!)

$$z = -1, 7, \pm j, \pm\sqrt{3}j, \pm\sqrt{2}j, \pm\sqrt{2}j$$

after observing we can factorise the polynomial.

Example 7   let $n = 10$, $a_0 = 10$, $a_{10} = 1$ and for $1 \le i \le 9$, $a_i = 0$. Then we have

$$z^{10} + 10 = 0$$

An application of de Moivre's theorem (refer to text on complex numbers for details) gives the following ten solutions

$$z = \left(10^{\frac{1}{10}}\right)\left(\cos\left(\left(\tfrac{2n+1}{10}\right)\pi\right) + j\sin\left(\left(\tfrac{2n+1}{10}\right)\pi\right)\right) \text{ for } n = 0,1,2,3,\ldots,9$$

Note that the value of $(10^{\frac{1}{10}})$ represents the single 'real' 10th root of 10 in the above expression, but also that all ten solutions of the equation are complex ones.

Although we often have discussion about polynomials of second, third or even tenth degree, these pale into insignificance when we consider the likes of polynomials of the 200th, the 1000th or even the *googol*th degree (where a *googol* is 10^{100}). A polynomial of the form

$$\sum_{i=0}^{googol} a_i z^i = 0$$

will have in general a *googol* roots. Of course our work might be simplified in those cases when most of the constants a_i are zero. The equation

$$z^{googol} + googol = 0 \text{ where } n = googol, a_0 = googol, a_{googol} = 1$$

with the other coefficients zero
has solutions

$$z = \left(googol^{\frac{1}{googol}} \right)\left(\cos\left(\left(\tfrac{2n+1}{googol}\right)\pi\right)\right) + j\sin\left(\left(\tfrac{2n+1}{googol}\right)\pi\right)$$

as n varies between 0 and *googol* − 1. Returning to our earlier discussion on the simple expression

$$x^x$$

we had noted that at least for real positive numbers we only generated one output for each individual value of x. Now that we are allowing for complex numbers this is no longer the case – writing the expression as

$$z^z$$

observe that unless z is an integer, multivalues are obtained (the expression is undefined when $z = 0$). The behaviour of these outputs is bizarre, and for negative integers alternate in sign while staying in real value. Thus when

$z = -5$, $z^z = -5^{-5} = -\frac{1}{3125}$ but when $z = -6$, $z^z = -6^{-6} = \frac{1}{46656}$

when $z = \frac{1}{4}$, z^z generates four possible values $\pm\frac{\sqrt{2}}{2}$ and $\pm\frac{\sqrt{2}j}{2}$

when $z = -\frac{1}{10}$, z^z generates ten values of the equation in Example 7 while if $z = \frac{-1}{googol}$, a *googol* possibilities are generated. Written out in full, this stirs the mind. From a seemingly straightforward expression with just one power level, by using the input value of $\frac{-1}{googol}$ we see that there are a total of

10000000000000000000000000000000000000000000000000000000000000000000000000000000000000000000000000000
possible outcomes!

If all this seems perplexing enough, just imagine how much more complicated things get when we consider an expression of the form

$$z_1^{z_2^{z_3 \cdots}}$$

where the power tower level extends to n levels and z_i $(i \leq 1 \leq n)$ are all complex numbers. Remember that even with a five-level power tower with real positive x domain we were generating nine distinct outputs. How many different outputs could we obtain for a fixed value of each z_i when $n = googol$?

What about measuring up?

Mathematics is filled with tiny details and fascinations that just cry out to be discovered. It is the very nature of the subject that can appeal to many with an eye for detail, including autistic individuals. Being able to solve a problem or simply ponder intriguing paradoxes that have no solution can be fun in its own right. For example, how long is the nearest table to you? How could you ever find out? You might say I would grab a ruler or tape measure. But this would only give you an approximation. Your eyesight can only see down to a certain level, say to the nearest millimetre. You will never know *exactly* how long it is, since you can keep dividing up a millimetre into smaller and smaller intervals. Besides, how accurate is the ruler or tape measure? The people who produce them may have no better eyesight than you! All we have done is take their word for it that it is as accurate as possible. But on a microscopic level, each ruler or tape measure is almost certainly a different length from another one, even if they both say otherwise. The same sort of thing could be said about asking someone what the time is. You look at your watch, sure. But is that accurate? You could check with the pips on the radio – surely that cannot be wrong? But even that cannot be *exactly* tuned to the correct time. Length and time intervals are examples of continuous data, they can only ever be approximated.

Why is the world the way it is?

There is another complication too. Our vision of the world is constantly of the past. When we see our friends in the same room as us, we are never seeing them as they are at that particular instant, but as they were in the recent past! Incredible though this may seem, this phenomenon can be explained by the fact that the speed of light is not infinite, and it takes time for the signals of their outlines to travel to your eyes to be registered by the brain into your field of view. But do not worry, we are only talking about millionths of a second, so your friends will not be able to nick your wallet in that time without you noticing (and you will not be able to do it to them either!). No framework of supposed events can be completely watertight. How do you know that the sun will rise in the east tomorrow morning, for example? The simple truth of the matter is that you do not know for *absolutely certain* that it will! You can say that it is extremely probable on past evidence perhaps to the odds of several quadrillion to one in your favour that it will, but you have no absolute proof. What if a sudden interstellar event such as a supernova shifted the Earth's orbit in the night and forced the sun to appear to rise in the west? Such a tiny probability of an event like this is so small it is normally neglected. But it is greater than zero, and this tiny detail is the sort of thing an autistic mind can pick up on! There will always also be other questions, such as why are we here at all and who or what made the universe, that we simply do not have answers to. The most we can hope to do is to observe the events of the world as we see them unfolding and try to adapt and be ready for what is likely to follow. Accessing the likelihood of an event and deciding how to plan for it if it occurs can be the foothold of a successful and fulfilling life for the individual.

Useful Addresses
and Further Reading

CARD – Center for Autism and Related Disorders
www.centerforautism.com

CCPD – Computer Centre for People with Disabilities
University of Westminster
72 Great Portland Street
London W1W 7NH
Tel: 020 7911 5808
www.wmin.ac.uk/ccpd

Children in Touch
c/o Thomley Centre Ltd
Menmarsh Road
Worminghall
Bucks HP18 9JZ
Tel: 01844 338696
kathy@childrenintouchtrust.co.uk

Circles Network
Potford's Dam Farm
Coventry Road
Cawston
Rugby CV23 9JP
Tel: 01788 816671
www.circlesnetwork.org.uk

DRC – Disability Rights Commission
DRC Helpline
Freepost MID02164
Stratford upon Avon
CV37 9BR
Tel: 08457 622633
www.drc-gb.org

Horizon Sports Club
anita_templar@hotmail.com

LEAP – London Early Autism Project
LEAP House
699 Fulham Road
London SW6 5UJ
Tel: 020 7736 6688
www.londonearlyautism.com

NCIL – National Centre for Independent Living
250 Kennington Lane
London SE11 5RD
Tel: 020 7585 1663
www.ncil.org.uk

PEACH – Parents for the Early Intervention of Autism in Children
The Brackens
London Road
Ascot
Berks SL5 8BE
Tel: 01344 882248
www.peach.org.uk

PECS – Picture Exchange Communication System
Pyramid Educational Consultants UK Ltd
Pavilion House
6 Old Steine
Brighton BN1 1EJ
Tel: 01273 609555
www.pecs.org.uk

RADAR – Royal Association for Disability and Rehabilitation
12 City Forum
250 City Road
London EC1V 8AF
Tel: 020 7250 3222
www.radar.org.uk

Skill – National Bureau for Students with Disabilities
Chapter House
18–20 Crucifix Lane
London SE1 3JW
Tel: 020 7450 0620
www.skill.org.uk

The National Autistic Society
393 City Road
London EC1V 1NG
Tel: 020 7833 2299
Autism Helpline: 0845 070 4004
www.nas.org.uk

Mesibov, G.B., Schopler, E. and Hearsey, K.A. (1994) *Structured Teaching.* New York: Plenum Books.
Son-Rise Programme. Kaufman, B.N. (1981) *A Miracle To Believe In.* New York: Ballantine Books.

Index